EQUIPPING HEALTH CARE LEADERS IN PAPUA NEW GUINEA

CAPACITY BUILDING FOR FUTURE HEALTH EXECUTIVES AND BETTER HEALTH OUTCOMES

FEBRUARY 2026

ASIAN DEVELOPMENT BANK

ADB

6 ADB Avenue, Mandaluyong City, 1550 Metro Manila, Philippines
Tel +63 2 8632 4444; Fax +63 2 8636 2444
www.adb.org

ISBN 978-92-9277-662-6 (print); 978-92-9277-663-3 (PDF); 978-92-9277-664-0 (ebook)
Publication Stock No. SPR260028-2
DOI: http://dx.doi.org/10.22617/SPR260028-2

Note:
In this publication, "$" refers to United States dollars.

Layout and design by Solveig Bang.

Contents

Figures and Box iv

Acknowledgments v

Abbreviations vi

Executive Summary vii

Background 1

Creation of Provincial Health Authorities 3

- Gaps in Leadership and Governance 4
- Asian Development Bank and Health in Papua New Guinea 7

Health Executive Leadership Development Program 10

- Need for Health Executive Leadership Training 10
- Delivering Health Executive Leadership Training 10
- Demanding, Face-to-Face, and Highly Context-Specific 14

Insights and Inspiration From the Training 16

- Need for a More Strategic Mindset 16
- Leaders as the Bridge from Policy to Action 17
- Everyone Can Teach ... and Learn 17
- Leadership, Management, and Governance in the Melanesian Context 18
- Overseas Study Tour 18

Beyond Theory to Practice: What Changed After the Training 22

- Direction and Momentum 23
- Working as a Team 23
- Improvement Mentality 24
- Communication Style 24
- Time and People Management 25
- New Network of Support 25

Graduate Projects 28

- Health Data Collection 28
- Clinical Waste Management 28
- Assets Registry 29
- Wellness Centers 29

Reflections and Recommendations 32

- Reflections 32
- Recommendations 34

Figures and Box

Figures

1 Papua New Guinea—Key Health Facts 1
2 Papua New Guinea Health Care Reforms Timeline 3
3 Middle Manager Development Workshops Program Training Topics 8
4 Health Executive Leadership Development Program 11
5 Core Skills of an Effective Health Executive 13
6 Study Tour Destinations 19
7 What Changed After the Leadership Training 22
8 Recommendations 34

Box

Training Effective Health System Managers 8

Acknowledgments

To those who championed and elicited interest in the program: Minister of Health Elias Kapavore, former Minister of Health Lino Tom, Acting National Department of Health Secretary Ken Wai, former National Department of Health Secretary Osborne Liko, Autonomous Region of Bougainville (North Solomon Province) Government former Acting Secretary of Health Clement Totavun, University of Papua New Guinea's School of Business & Public Policy and School of Medicine & Health Sciences, Divine Word University's Faculty of Medicine & Health, Port Moresby General Hospital Chief Executive Officer Paki Molumi, and the Chief Executive Officers of Provincial Health Authorities of Papua New Guinea (PNG): Central, Simbu (Chimbu), Eastern Highlands, East New Britain, East Sepik, Enga, Gulf, Hela, Jiwaka, Madang, Manus, Milne Bay, Morobe, National Capital District, New Ireland, Oro (Northern), Sandaun (West Sepik), Southern Highlands, West New Britain, Western Highlands, and Western (Fly River).

To nongovernment organization and institutional partners, who nominated participants and provided guest lecturers: Catholic Church Health Services, Christian Health Services, Australian Doctors International, Femili PNG, Oxfam International, Rotarians Against Malaria, Santos Foundation, Tabubil Hospital (Ok Tedi Mining Limited), University of Melbourne (Australia), and Vital Strategies for Bloomberg Philanthropies Data for Health (D4H) Initiative.

To government partners, who facilitated timely provision of passports and visas for participants: Australian Department of Foreign Affairs & Trade, PNG Department of Foreign Affairs, and PNG Immigration & Citizenship Authority.

To the hosts of the international study tour: Malaysia (Malaysian Society for Quality in Health; Singapore (Singapore Changi General Hospital, Singapore Health Promotion Board, International SOS Medical Logistics Hub); and Australia (Townsville University Hospital, James Cook University Medical School, Northern Territory Health Services & Royal Darwin Hospital, Northern Territory Danila Dilba Aboriginal Health Services).

To the course facilitators of the PNG Health Services Sector Development Program (HSSDP), in particular HSSDP Human Resource Development Specialist Peter Baran, who developed content, facilitates delivery, coordinates travel and accommodation arrangements locally and abroad, and delivers lectures.

To the 32 interviewees for this report, and to HSSDP Project Manager Rob Akers, for facilitating the interviews.

Abbreviations

CCHS	Catholic Church Health Services
CHS	Christian Health Services
DOH	Department of Health
DWU	Divine Word University
HELDP	Health Executive Leadership Development Program
HSSDP	Health Services Sector Development Program
NDOH	National Department of Health
NGO	nongovernment organization
PHA	Provincial Health Authority
PNG	Papua New Guinea
RPHSDP	Rural Primary Health Services Delivery Project
UPNG	University of Papua New Guinea
WHO	World Health Organization

Executive Summary

In Papua New Guinea (PNG), the Provincial Health Authorities (PHA) Act 2007 created the foundation of the health system at the provincial level, with decentralization intended to bring the organization of health care closer to the people served and to resolve issues of fragmentation of health services delivery. While the formation of PHAs addressed a need to bring health system governance and management nearer to the population, the limited investment in management and leadership skills has hampered progress. From the first three pilot PHAs set up in 2009, through to the last in 2019, it became increasingly clear that there was a leadership vacuum that was contributing to the sluggish establishment and operationalization of the PHAs' structures, functions and policies.

Through intensive residencies culminating in an overseas study tour, the Health Executive Leadership Development Program has trained 110 executives drawn from the Department of Health and most of the country's provinces.

As part of its decades-long and ongoing support to PNG for health systems strengthening, the Asian Development Bank (ADB) recognized these limitations and included investment in this capacity gap under the Health Services Sector Development Program (HSSDP), which was approved in 2018, with joint financing from ADB and the Australian Government. The program developed leadership training for both middle management and executives. Through intensive residencies culminating in an overseas study tour, the Health Executive Leadership Development Program (HELDP) has trained 110 executives drawn from the Department of Health and most of the country's provinces.

The program content, developed by leadership experts with extensive experience in the country, combined theory and practical implementation, tailored to PNG and the wider Melanesian cultural context. It was delivered using a face-to-face, problem-based learning modality. Program graduates, their managers and other stakeholders report that the program has been transformative, leading to visibly improved leadership confidence, decision-making, and organizational performance. At an institutional level, there is evidence of better coordination within PHAs and stronger alignment with national health strategies. The rollout of HELDP in PNG offers useful insights to other developing countries with complex health challenges and health services delivery constraints.

This report examines the impact of HELDP, draws out the leadership program's successes and lessons learned, and captures the experiences of a variety of stakeholders. Data were gathered through interviews with 32 stakeholders, including 17 HELDP graduates (7 women, 10 men), facilitators, health care providers, government officials, and funders.

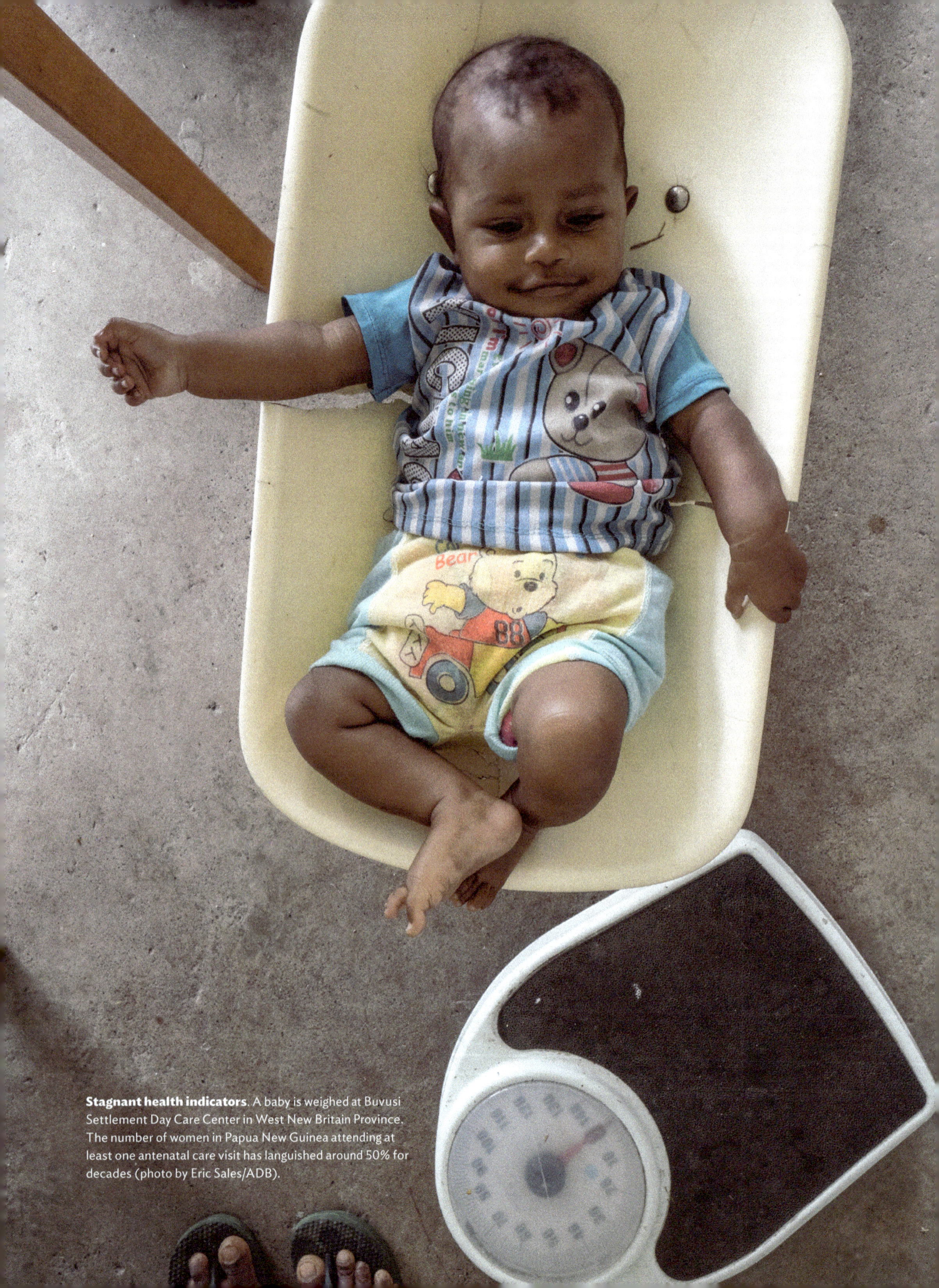

Stagnant health indicators. A baby is weighed at Buvusi Settlement Day Care Center in West New Britain Province. The number of women in Papua New Guinea attending at least one antenatal care visit has languished around 50% for decades (photo by Eric Sales/ADB).

Background

In Papua New Guinea (PNG), health services delivery operates under several severe constraints, including vulnerability to natural hazards, security risks, and large areas of the country that are remote and accessible only on foot, or by boat or aircraft. Lack of investment in health facility infrastructure and human resources for health, as well as inefficient health information and medical supply distribution systems create additional hurdles to managing health care delivery and to universal health care coverage.[1]

In Papua New Guinea, health services delivery operates under several severe constraints. Key health indicators are stagnant or even deteriorating.

Key health indicators are stagnant or even deteriorating. The number of women attending the WHO-recommended minimum of four antenatal visits, was 54.9% between 2003 and 2006, but fell to 49% in the period from 2011 to 2018.[2] From 2019 to 2024, coverage was even worse, with only 29% of pregnant women receiving at least four antenatal visits.[2] Diphtheria-tetanus-pertussis (DTP3) immunization coverage among one-year-olds fell from 59% in 2000 to 42% in 2024.[3] While the number of health workers per 10,000 population nationally improved between 2020 and 2024, from 9 per 10,000 in both 2020 and 2021, to 14 in 2024, this is still well below the 2025 national target of 18 and the 2030 target of 20 per 10,000 population (footnote 2).

Figure 1: Papua New Guinea—Key Health Facts

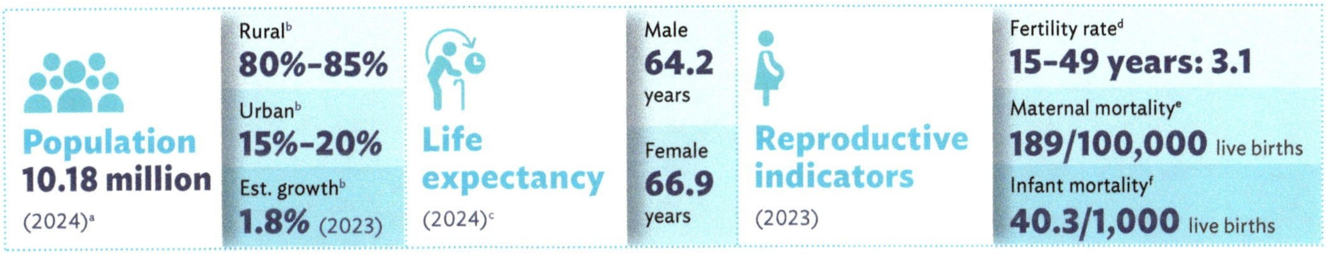

a. National Statistical Office of Papua New Guinea. November 2025. 2024 National Population Census.
b. World Bank Data. 2023. Urban population (% of total population) – Papua New Guinea.
c. National Statistical Office of Papua New Guinea. 2024. Health.
d. World Bank Group Data. Fertility rate, total (births per woman) - Papua New Guinea. 2023.
e. United Nations Population Fund. Papua New Guinea Population 2025.
f. UNICEF Data. Monitoring the situation of women and children. Papua New Guinea.

[1] World Health Organization (WHO). 2019. *Health in Transition: Papua New Guinea*. Manila.

[2] PNG National Department of Health. October 2025. *2024 Sector Performance Annual Review.*

[3] WHO data. Diphtheria-tetanus-pertussis (DTP3) immunization coverage among 1 year olds (%). Official estimate updated 15 July 2025.

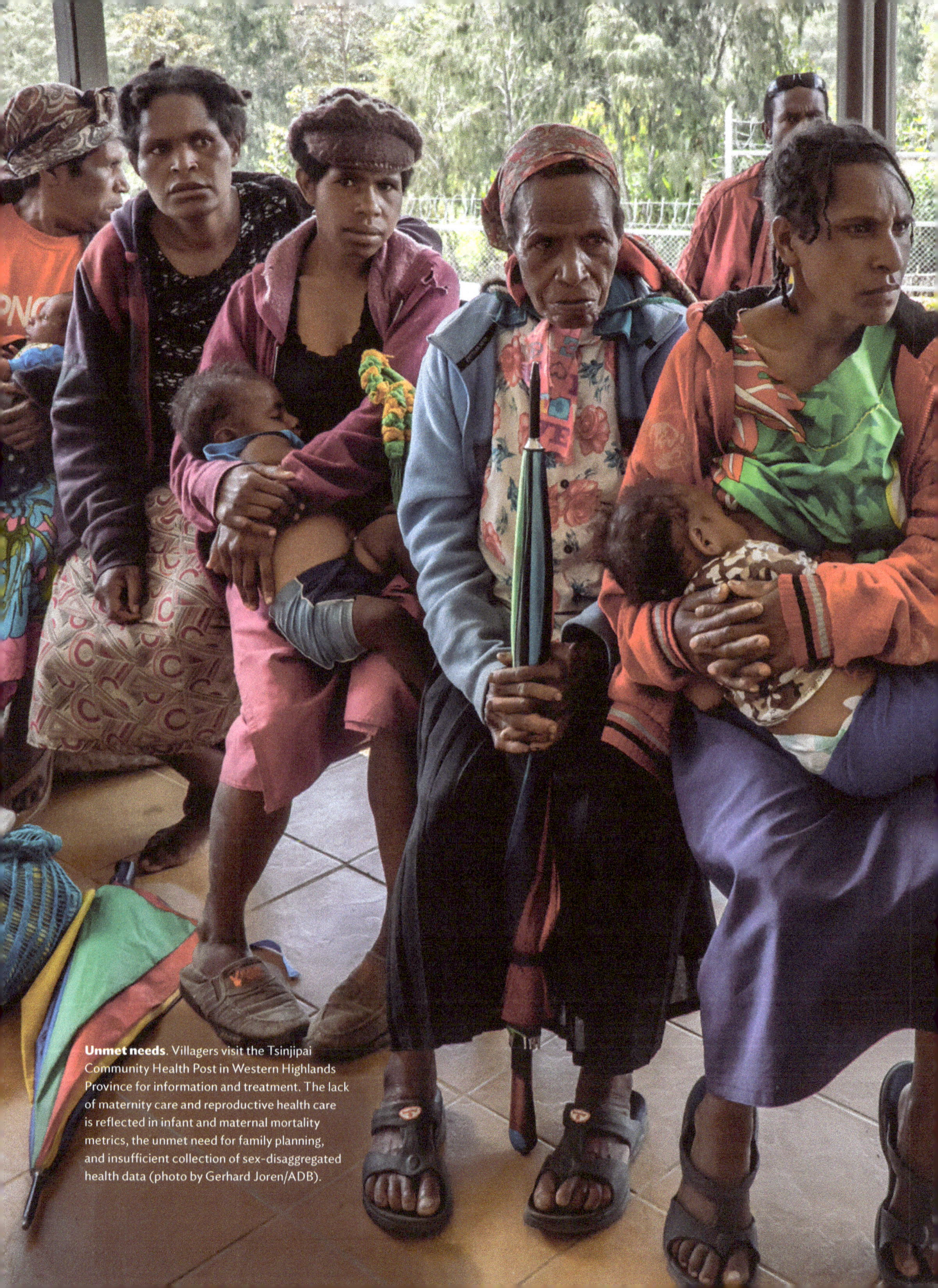

Unmet needs. Villagers visit the Tsinjipai Community Health Post in Western Highlands Province for information and treatment. The lack of maternity care and reproductive health care is reflected in infant and maternal mortality metrics, the unmet need for family planning, and insufficient collection of sex-disaggregated health data (photo by Gerhard Joren/ADB).

Creation of Provincial Health Authorities

The Provincial Health Authorities ensure that the overarching vision of the National Health Strategy is realized in health service provision.

Since its independence in 1975, PNG has implemented a series of health care reforms, with the National Health Administration Act 1997 determining the structure of the health system, and the Provincial Health Authorities (PHA) Act 2007 (amended in 2013 and 2023) tasking PHAs with health service delivery at all levels, from provincial hospitals to community health posts, and managing their own budgets. This decentralization was intended to make the health care system more responsive to population needs and resolve issues of fragmentation of health services delivery.[4]

The 2007 act enabled the creation of a PHA for each of the country's 22 provincial divisions, including the Autonomous Region of Bougainville and the National Capital District of Port Moresby. The process began in 2009 with the formation of three PHAs, growing to nine by 2016, and with a full rollout by 2019, with each PHA overseeing the planning, management, and delivery of health care services, supervised by a board of directors appointed by the National Executive Council on the recommendation of the provincial government.

The PHAs are the mechanisms through which the country's health policy is implemented. They ensure that the overarching vision of the PNG National Health Strategy is realized in health service provision, along with the Sustainable Development Goals, which target universal health coverage by 2030.[5] The decentralization of responsibility to the PHAs has not been well planned, either in terms of policy or implementation. Limited human resources and capacity at the managerial level have hindered evidence-based decision-making. This in turn affects planning, budgeting, and monitoring, and also contributes to low staff morale, inequitable service distribution, and preventable morbidity and mortality.

Figure 2: Papua New Guinea Health Care Reforms Timeline

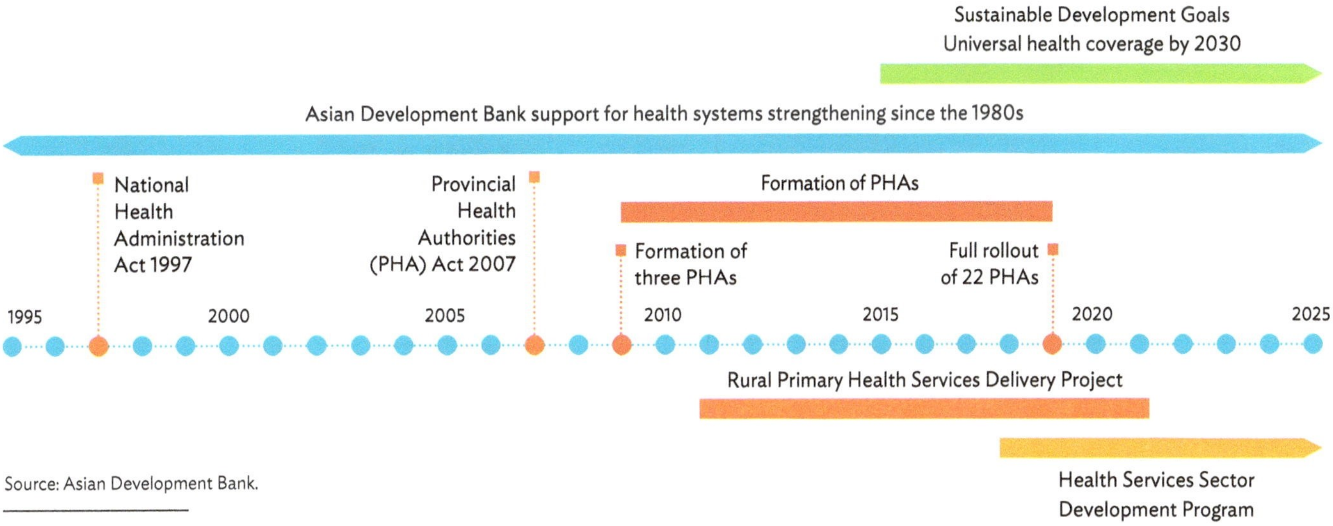

Source: Asian Development Bank.

[4] Government of PNG. 2015. Independent Review. Provincial Health Authority. Management and Structures. Port Moresby.

[5] Government of Papua New Guinea. National Health Plan 2021–2030 Volume 1: Policies and Strategies, 2021; United Nations Department of Economic and Social Affairs. Sustainable Development Goals. SDG 3: Ensure healthy lives and promote well-being for all at all ages; and the Independent State of Papua New Guinea National Strategic Plan Taskforce. Papua New Guinea Vision 2050. 2010.

GAPS IN LEADERSHIP AND GOVERNANCE

The formation of PHAs aimed to bolster health system governance and management structures, and bring the health system closer to the population. However, a severe lack of human resources within the health system, including staff with management and leadership skills, has hampered progress. From the first three pilot PHAs set up in 2009 to the establishment of the last in 2019, it became increasingly clear that there were significant gaps in leadership that contributed to sluggish implementation.

Significant gaps in leadership contributed to sluggish PHA implementation.

These gaps are indicative of a lack of investment in leadership training in the health sector. There are established training pathways for community health workers—typically run by church organizations that deliver much of the primary care in rural areas—as well as for nurses and midwives, through numerous schools of nursing. The University of Papua New Guinea (UPNG) and Divine Word University (DWU) offer medical and public health degree programs, and DWU also offers an undergraduate degree in health services management. However, the only postgraduate management training available in PNG's tertiary sector is not specific to the health sector. Meanwhile, health system management training abroad is expensive and not sufficiently relevant to the PNG context.

Career limitations

The typical career trajectory of health system leaders means that chief executive officer positions are usually filled by physicians who have risen to the top of their clinical career ladder. There have been scant opportunities for these technically highly skilled clinicians to undergo management training or to acquire the strategic skills for health systems leadership. Professionals from other segments of the health system have even more limited opportunities to demonstrate their leadership potential.

As a result, there are significant gaps in how PNG's health system is managed, including leadership capacity, governance, health financing, data management, and accountability systems. There are not enough adequately trained leaders, at either the provincial or the district level, to translate policy into effective service delivery. Coordination between the national, provincial, and facility levels is weak, often leading to resource allocation inefficiency, service delivery delays, and ultimately poor health outcomes, especially in rural areas.

Shortcomings in accountability

By the early 2020s, this skills gap was manifesting itself in poorly managed health services, with wide variation in the performance of PHAs. It also became apparent through the extremely low levels of data reporting to the Department of Health (DOH), despite routine reporting being mandated under the governing National Health Administration Act 1997. Few PHAs were fully meeting their data-reporting duties, which in turn severely undermined the DOH's ability to conduct evidence-based health services planning.

While the PHAs had a common regulatory framework and faced similar challenges, there was no opportunity for the senior leadership of PHAs to meet, compare experiences and collectively raise issues with the DOH.

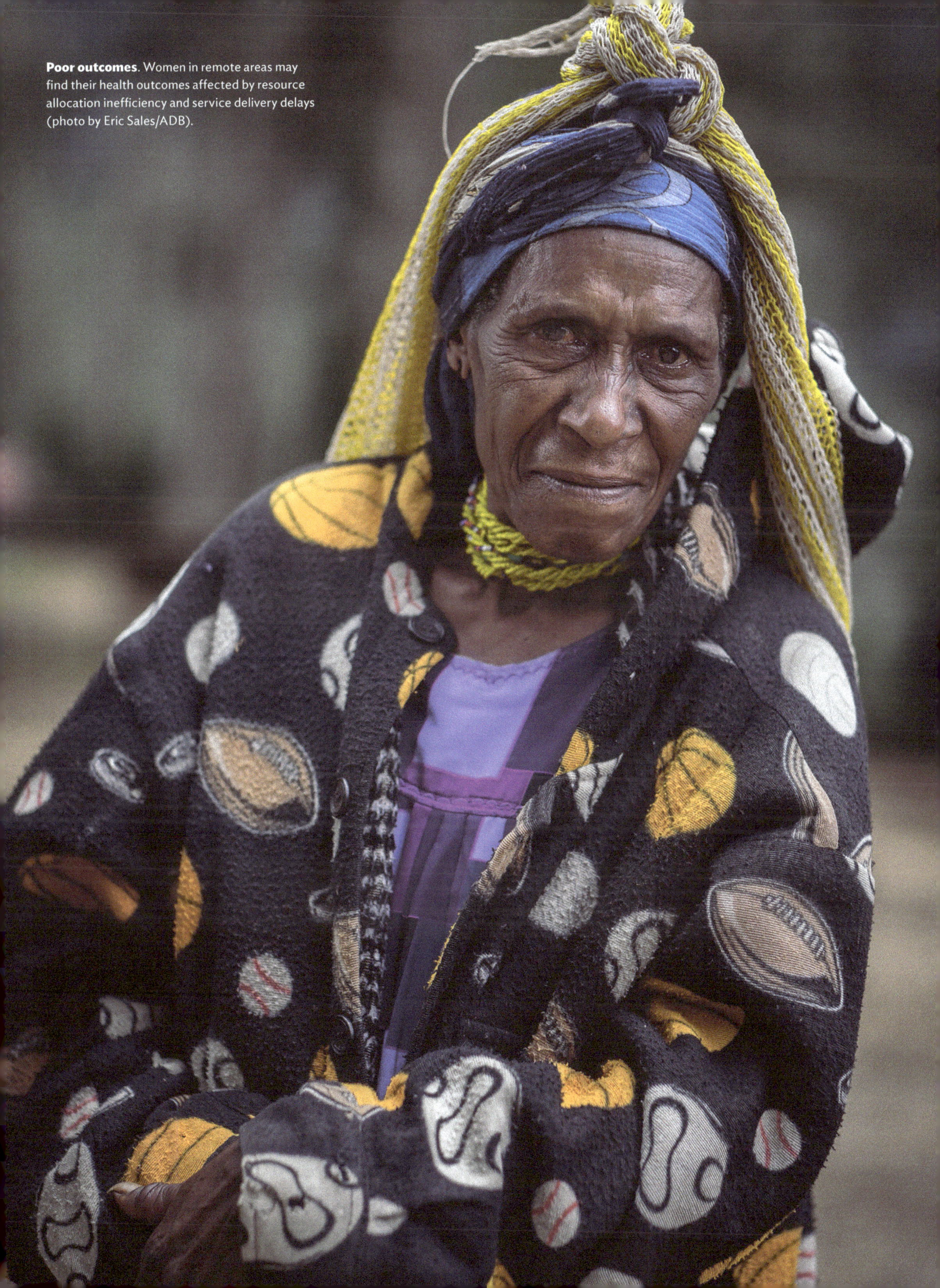

Poor outcomes. Women in remote areas may find their health outcomes affected by resource allocation inefficiency and service delivery delays (photo by Eric Sales/ADB).

Weak supervision structures

The skills gap has affected national health system management and was apparent among provincial senior management, such as the PHA executive leadership teams, as well as middle management, including those responsible for district health services delivery. This undermined efforts to improve the health system through infrastructure development. Without effective supervision and management, new hospitals and clinics either operate at suboptimal levels or—worse—may not even open at all, due to a lack of appropriate staffing and medical supplies.

Without effective supervision and management, new hospitals and clinics either operate at suboptimal levels or—worse—may not even open at all.

Women's low representation in sector leadership

Although women comprise half of the health care workforce in PNG, they are grossly underrepresented in the leadership ranks of the health system, part of a broader trend of female exclusion from decision-making roles, including in government at all levels.[6] Across the 21 PHAs and the Bougainville Department of Health, there are only two permanently appointed female chief executives, one female acting chief executive, nine female directors and eight female district health managers.

The low number of women in key leadership and decision-making roles at all levels is influenced by prevailing gender norms.[7] This gender disparity is recognized as a significant barrier to social development.[8] It also mirrors the gender inequalities in the health system overall, whereby men have more access to health care than women.[9] The lack of maternity care and reproductive health care is reflected in both infant and maternal mortality metrics, the unmet need for family planning, and insufficient gender disaggregation of health data (footnote 9).

The country's National Public Service Gender Equity & Social Inclusion (GESI) Policy aims to safeguard gender equality and social inclusion in the workplace.[10] The government's Action Plan for Implementing Gender Equality and Social Inclusion Across the National Public Service outlines strategies to encourage more women into the national public service, including sponsorship for and mentoring of women identified as having the potential to fill leadership roles (footnote 10). However, there has been little progress in enforcing the policy or strategies.[11]

These challenges of worsening health indicators, declining access and utilization, poorly managed health facilities and services, and failing data systems are only set to worsen, as the population continues to grow, and the double burden of communicable and lifestyle diseases increases.

---

[6] United Nations Population Fund in Papua New Guinea. N.d. Gender equality and women's empowerment.

[7] Australian Government Department of Foreign Affairs and Trade. Papua New Guinea–Australia Health Partnership Strategy 2024–2034.

[8] Australian High Commission Papua New Guinea. Feature Story: Breaking the Barrier: Gender Equality in Papua New Guinea's Health Sector.

[9] Dere S. The Borgen project. 22 July 2021. Women's Health in Papua New Guinea.

[10] Government of Papua New Guinea Department of Personnel Management. N.d. National Public Service Gender Equity & Social Inclusion (GESI) Policy: "Rise up, Step up, Speak up".

[11] Second Additional Financing of Health Services Sector Development Program (RRP PNG 51035). Sector Assessment (Summary): Health.

In 2022, there were 12,190 new cases of cancer reported, of which 6,801 were among women and 5,389 among men. In the same year, there were 7,200 deaths due to cancer (3,926 among women and 3,274 among men.) The top three cancers ranked by cases were breast, cervix/uteri, and lip/oral cavity for women; and prostate, lip/oral cavity, and liver for men. The risk of dying from cancer before the age of 75 years was 12.4% for women and 11.8% for men. The top three cancers ranked by deaths were breast, cervix/uteri, and liver for women, and liver, lung, and prostate for men.[12]

ASIAN DEVELOPMENT BANK AND HEALTH IN PAPUA NEW GUINEA

The Asian Development Bank (ADB) has been supporting PNG's health systems strengthening efforts since the 1980s. Investment in leadership and management began under the Rural Primary Health Services Delivery Project (RPHSDP) from 2011 to 2021, coinciding with the formation of PHAs, and—building on the achievements and lessons of that initiative—the Health Services Sector Development Program (HSSDP), which began in 2018 and is ongoing.[13]

The Asian Development Bank has been supporting Papua New Guinea's health systems strengthening efforts since the 1980s.

The HSSDP is a $266 million project under the DOH, co-financed by ADB and the Australian Government. It supports health systems strengthening through the refurbishment of existing health care infrastructure, construction of new facilities, health policy and planning reform, and capacity building. Under the RPHSDP, the DOH began addressing the management skills gap, bringing in a health management expert with extensive experience in PNG and other developing country settings to design and run management skills training workshops for PHA and district health managers. Managers from eight provinces completed the training under the RPHSDP, and the training continued under the HSSDP, expanding to the rest of the country (see Box: Training Effective Health System Managers).

Through interactions with hundreds of trainees, facilitators gained useful insights into managers' workplace dynamics and conditions in PHAs and into the two church organizations responsible for service delivery, Christian Health Services (CHS) and Catholic Church Health Services (CCHS). It became clear, for example, that participants were not aware of documents that were directly related to their work, including the 2021-2030 National Health Plan and National Health Service Standards, various national health policies, and the relevant provincial strategies, policies and plans.

There was also generally limited district-level planning that was aligned with PHA priorities, and there was a lack of guidance for PHA organizational structure, human resources policies, and information sharing. Clearly there was a need to modernize health system organization and to move on from the 1970s command-and-control approach. This led to the decision to launch a separate program for the executive level and informed the program's content to address these gaps.

---

[12] Global Cancer Observatory. 2022. Papua New Guinea.

[13] Asian Development Bank. Papua New Guinea: Rural Primary Health Services Delivery Project. Sovereign Project 41509-013; ADB. Papua New Guinea: Health Services Sector Development Program, Subprogram 1. Sovereign Project 51035-001; and ADB. Papua New Guinea: Health Services Sector Development Program (Second Additional Financing). Sovereign Project 51035-006.

Box: Training Effective Health System Managers

The Middle Manager Development Workshops Program began in 2018 and, by late 2025, had trained more than 1,300 health system managers (about half of them women) in every province. Most of the participants had not previously received any formal management or supervisory training.

Delivered over 5 consecutive days, the training was designed to give an intensive, rapid and broad overview of the key aspects of managing a team, a work program and oneself, and to improve managers' performance. The program's objectives were to empower managers to understand their key functional roles and the difference between management and leadership. It covered how to effectively build and maintain a high-performance work team, and how to apply a range of management techniques and practices (box figure).

Figure 3: Middle Manager Development Workshops Program Training Topics

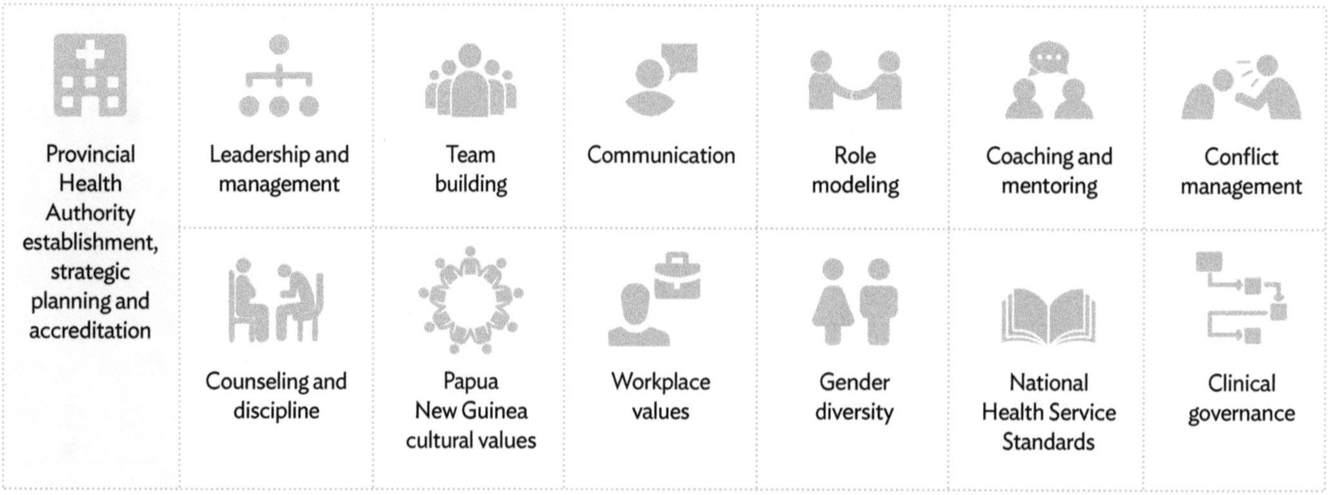

Source: Asian Development Bank.

There were group exercises based on case studies and problem-solving, for example on motivating staff, resolving conflict in the workplace, PHA performance on maternal and child health indicators, gender diversity, and PNG cultural values. The training received high appraisal ratings and positive feedback from participants, as well as ideas for improvement, which were used to refine subsequent training sessions.

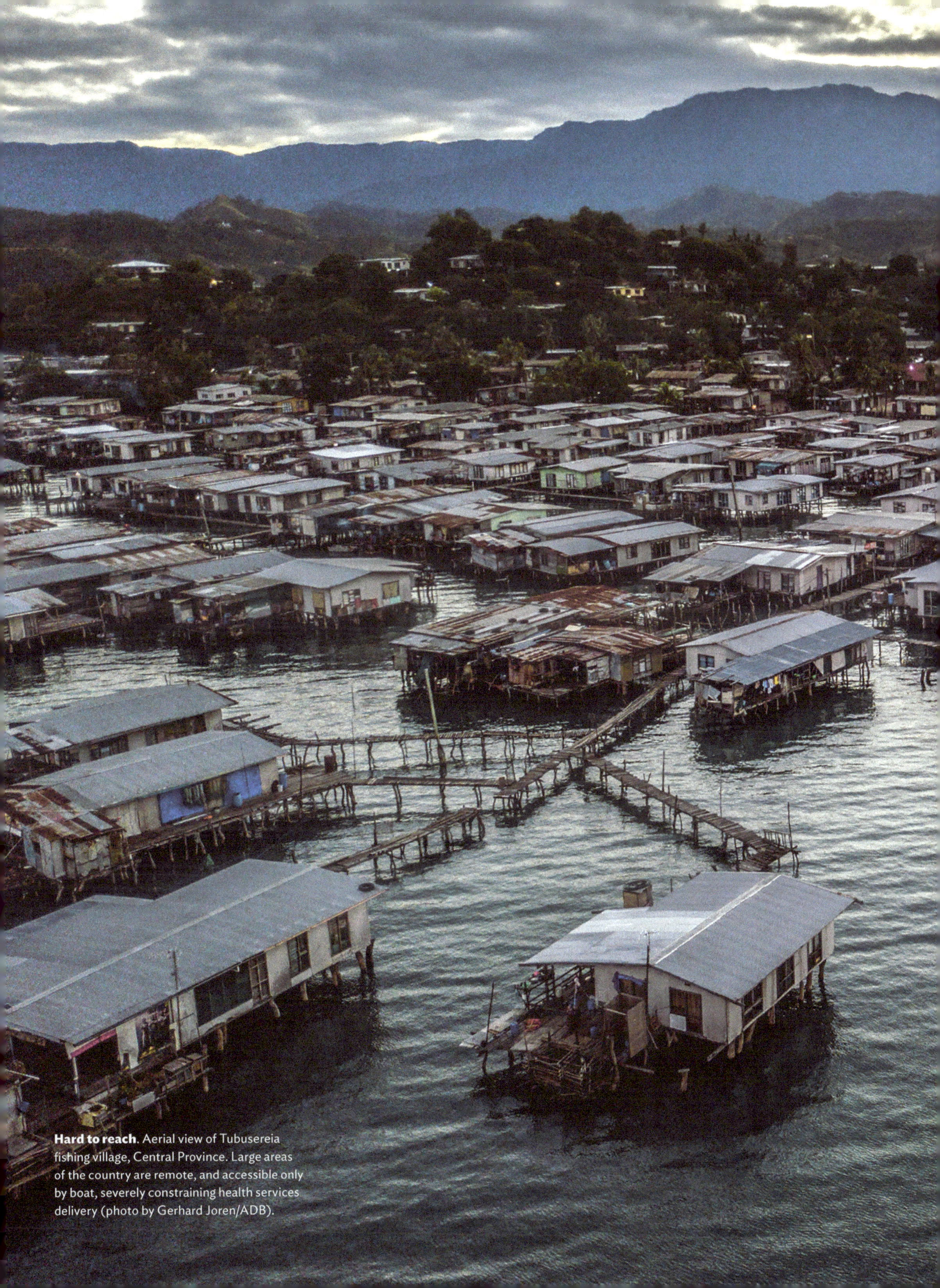

Hard to reach. Aerial view of Tubusereia fishing village, Central Province. Large areas of the country are remote, and accessible only by boat, severely constraining health services delivery (photo by Gerhard Joren/ADB).

Health Executive Leadership Development Program

While training hundreds of middle managers under the HSSDP, it became increasingly clear that executives also needed support. Having been disrupted by the COVID-19 pandemic, in early 2023, the HSSDP launched the Health Executive Leadership Development Program (HELDP), inducting its first cohort of 33 trainees in March that year.

NEED FOR HEALTH EXECUTIVE LEADERSHIP TRAINING

The rationale for HELDP is that the transition from a senior manager to an organizational executive leader is more than just a promotion. It requires a significant change process across all aspects of leadership, management and organizational development, from how executives manage themselves to how they interact with others, and ultimately how they engage the broader organization in which they work.

A new building is not a health facility until it can be properly staffed and managed.

As HELDP is nested within a larger project focused on the refurbishment and construction of health care facilities, it is tempting to think of it as a less tangible endeavor. Unlike the opening of a new clinic, the graduation of a new health leader does not present an opportunity for ribbon cutting and public celebration. However, a new building is not a health facility until it can be properly staffed and managed. Even then, it cannot effectively contribute to the broader goal of improved population health unless it is part of a well-run health system with leaders adept at strategic thinking and capable of long-term vision. At approximately $16,500 per trainee, the course is relatively expensive. However, this is seen by the DOH and HSSDP management as a long-term investment whose impact may only be evident in 3–5 years.

DELIVERING HEALTH EXECUTIVE LEADERSHIP TRAINING

The HELDP curriculum, designed in collaboration with the two universities—UPNG and DWU—consists of three 2-week residential training sessions. Each 2-week module occurs in a calendar quarter, and the course is completed within a year. The course (Figure 4) is held on the UPNG campus in Port Moresby, and culminates in a final session comprising a 1-week residential workshop and a 10-day overseas study tour. It adopts a blended model comprising academic learning, mentoring, and field-based projects. This enables trainees to immediately implement what they have learnt in between the training periods, and to begin improving health service efficiency and leadership accountability.

Figure 4: Health Executive Leadership Development Program

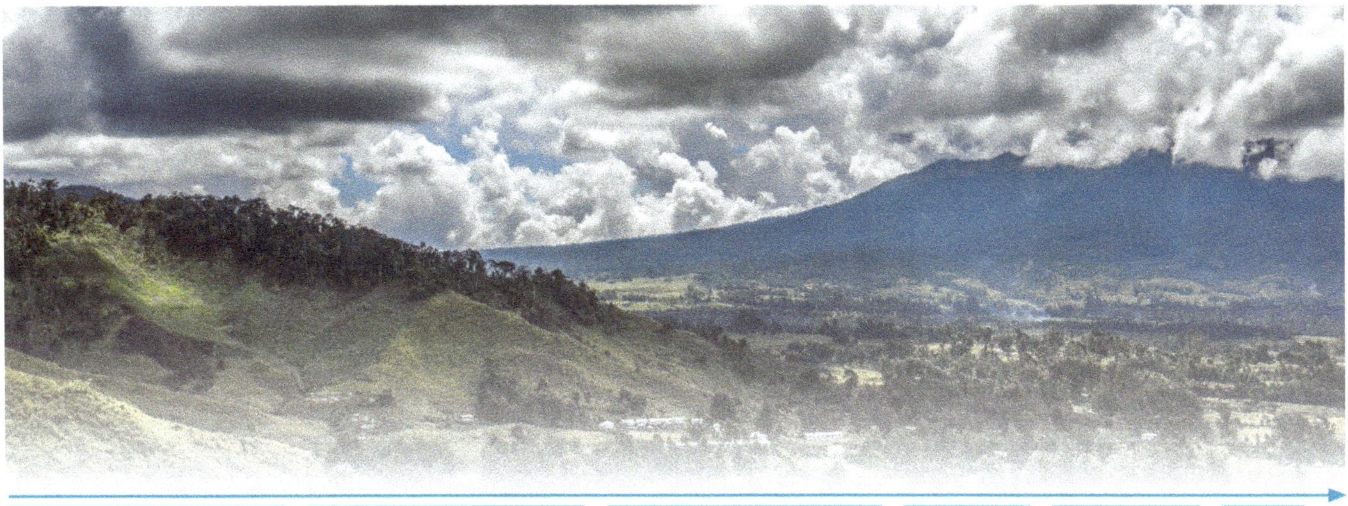

2 WEEKS | 2 WEEKS | 2 WEEKS | 1 WEEK | 10 DAYS

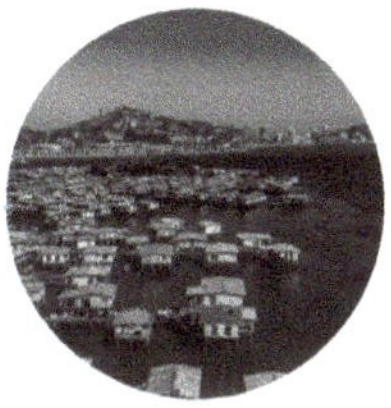

1

1st Residential Workshop

Future of Papua New Guinea Health

- Health planning.
- Corporate and clinical governance.
- Clinical risk management.
- Health data analytics, interpretation and policy implementation.
- Dealing with competing priorities.

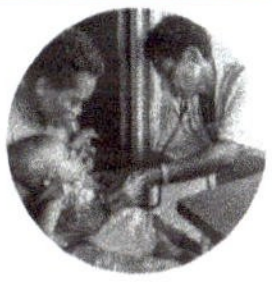

2

2nd Residential Workshop

Managing Yourself and Influencing Others

- Understanding the self in leadership and management.
- Emotional intelligence for leaders.
- Dealing with challenging people.
- Coaching, mentoring and motivation for high-performing teams.
- Gender, diversity and sensitivity issues.

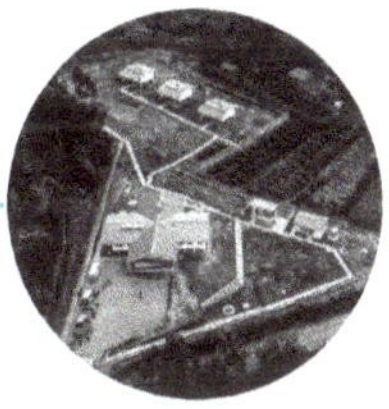

3

3rd Residential Workshop

Executing Leadership and Strategic Management

- Leadership, management, and health sector complexity.
- Political, shareholder and stakeholder management.
- Finance, legal, risk, and resource management.
- Marketing, promotion, presentation, and media.
- Communication and conflict resolution.

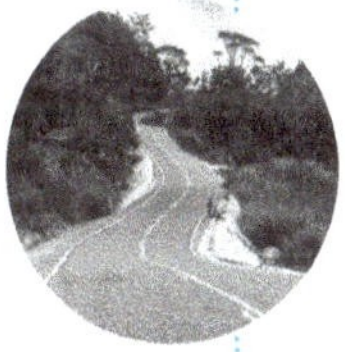

4

4th Residential Workshop

Leading for Organizational Results

- Managing operational costs.
- Change agent skills and change simulation.
- Customer/patient issues.
- Executive leadership perspectives.
- Future workforce perspectives.

Study tour

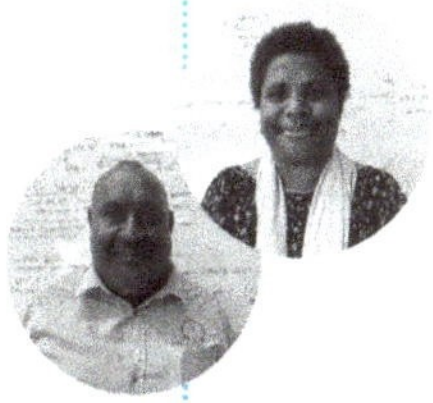

Individual project presentations

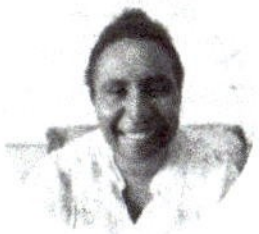

Each 2-week module occurs in a calendar quarter, and the course is completed within a year.

Across all four workshops

- Keynote speakers: Minister of Health, Secretary for Health, other senior leadership.
- Individual project consultation.
- Individual coaching and mentoring.

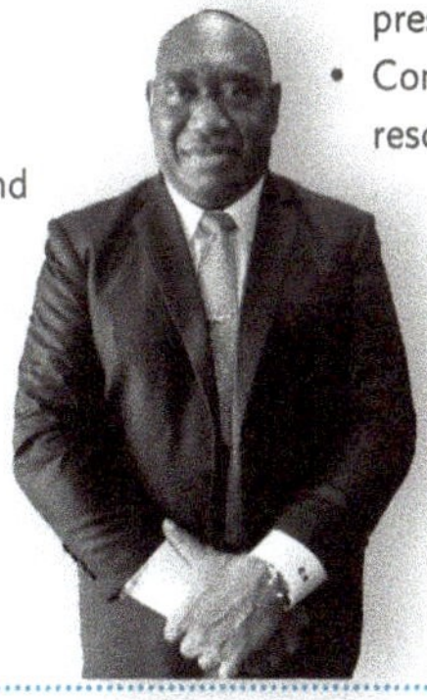

"Complementing infrastructure with good health leadership is fundamentally important."

Elias Kapavore
Minister for Health , Government of Papua New Guinea

Source: Asian Development Bank.

Selection process

Trainees are nominated by their supervisors or colleagues. Applications are then vetted by the secretary for health, the HSSDP manager, a human resources development expert, and faculty of UPNG and DWU. The trainees hold senior and middle management positions in the NDOH, PHAs, major hospitals, and the two church organizations, as well as in nongovernment organizations (NGOs) in the health sector. The selection process ensures that trainees are already sufficiently highly educated and experienced to benefit from the course, and are either already in executive roles, or clearly show leadership potential. The cohorts comprise a mix of trainees, including some who are in junior roles but performing key roles in which they also need to develop leadership and management skills.

The selection process ensures that trainees are already sufficiently highly educated and experienced to benefit from the course.

Course delivery

The course facilitators are drawn from both PNG and abroad, and there are eminent guest speakers, such as the minister of health. Faculty from both universities contributed to curriculum development, and are engaged in the delivery of modules and facilitation of in-class discussion. There is a strong focus on group work, case study-based learning and active involvement by all trainees. There are also individual assessments and tailored coaching. All trainees are required to complete an individual project that brings about a needed change within their organization, guided by one-to-one mentoring from university faculty.

As of the end of 2025, three cohorts had completed the training, for a total of 110 participants (46 women and 64 men). They came from almost every province in the country and worked in a wide variety of settings. A fourth cohort of 16 participants (9 male, 7 female) has begun training, with graduation scheduled for late 2026. The cost of the basic training was borne by the HSSDP for the first three cohorts, and the fourth cohort trainees are being financed by their institutions, evidence that the value of the course is recognized, and a testament to the high regard in which the program is held.

Expected outcomes

The desired result of the training is leaders who can exercise disciplined thinking, prioritize competing demands on resources, look objectively at returns on investment, and present strong evidence for their decisions. They can collaborate as part of the senior leadership team, manage competing priorities, and inspire their staff.

The purpose of the training is to create a pool of eligible applicants for senior leadership positions in the NDOH, the PHAs, and across the major health service providers, with the core job skills necessary for performance at an executive level (Figure 5). Another of the program's key aims is to increase diversity in the composition of the PNG health sector leadership, particularly ensuring more women and people with disabilities are better represented in leadership roles.

Figure 5: Core Skills of an Effective Health Executive

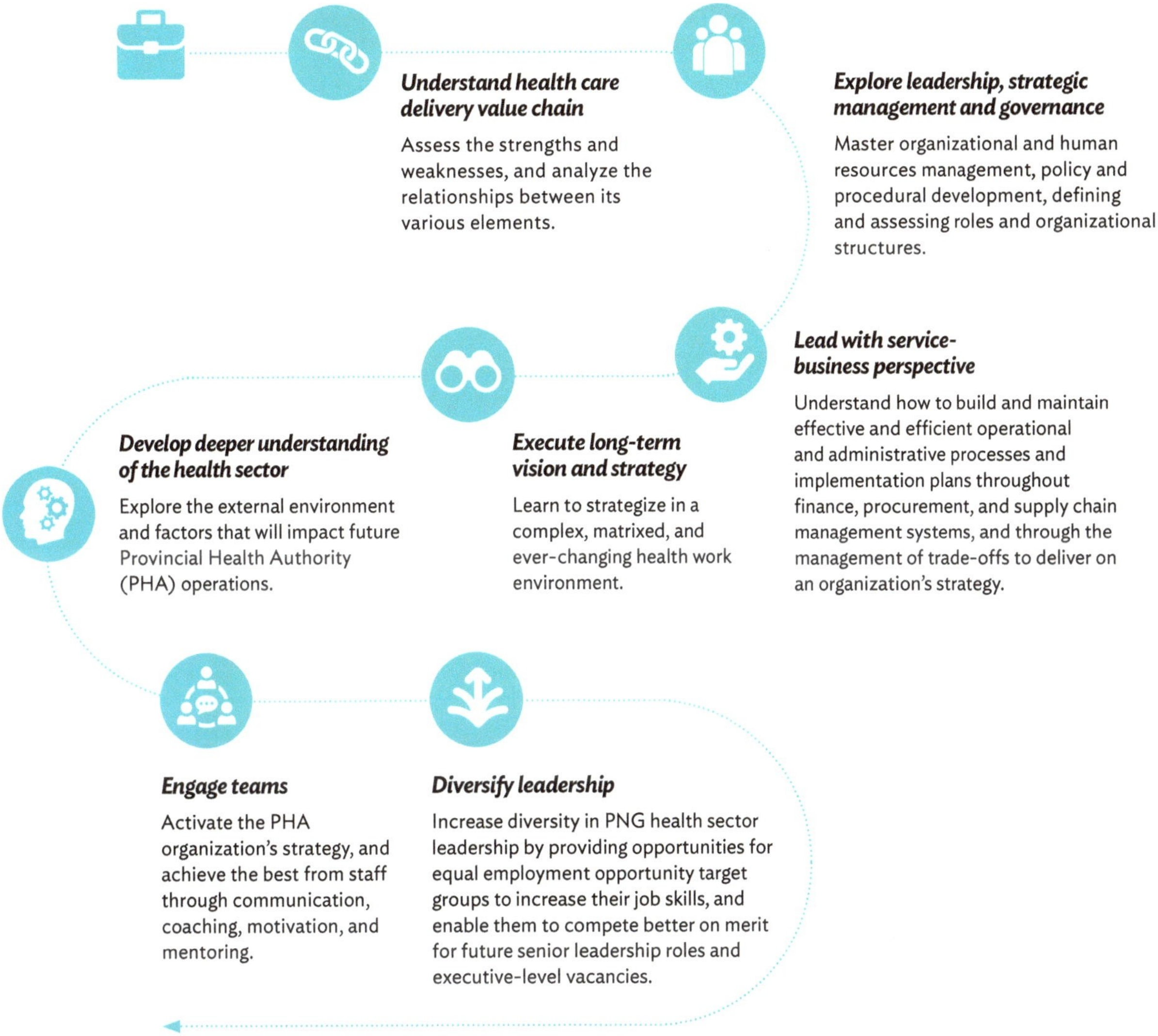
Understand health care delivery value chain
Assess the strengths and weaknesses, and analyze the relationships between its various elements.
Explore leadership, strategic management and governance
Master organizational and human resources management, policy and procedural development, defining and assessing roles and organizational structures.
Lead with service-business perspective
Understand how to build and maintain effective and efficient operational and administrative processes and implementation plans throughout finance, procurement, and supply chain management systems, and through the management of trade-offs to deliver on an organization's strategy.
Execute long-term vision and strategy
Learn to strategize in a complex, matrixed, and ever-changing health work environment.
Develop deeper understanding of the health sector
Explore the external environment and factors that will impact future Provincial Health Authority (PHA) operations.
Engage teams
Activate the PHA organization's strategy, and achieve the best from staff through communication, coaching, motivation, and mentoring.
Diversify leadership
Increase diversity in PNG health sector leadership by providing opportunities for equal employment opportunity target groups to increase their job skills, and enable them to compete better on merit for future senior leadership roles and executive-level vacancies.

Source: National Department of Health Fast Track 12-Month Health Executive Leadership Development Program, 2023 - 2024

HELDP differs from traditional university programs because of its applied, competency-based, and field-oriented design. Unlike academic degree programs that generally focus only on theory and research, HELDP combines executive education, mentoring, and experiential learning. It also emphasizes inter-sectoral collaboration and systems thinking, skills that are not necessarily taught in regular management or public health degrees. HELDP also offers university faculty an opportunity to engage with the health sector in new ways, giving them a better understanding of the dynamics and challenges of working life for executives in the PHAs and other parts of the health system.

DEMANDING, FACE-TO-FACE, AND HIGHLY CONTEXT-SPECIFIC

Traveling within PNG is expensive and air travel is the only way to reach the capital from most provinces. A significant portion of the program budget was spent on the logistics of getting trainees from across the country to Port Moresby, and accommodating them for 2 weeks at a time on the UPNG campus, as well as on the overseas study tour. These outlays have to be weighed against the impact of the face-to-face modality. Graduates were taken out of their daily surroundings and compelled to focus on the task at hand, without distractions from their regular job commitments. Trainees' absence from work also created an expectation among their managers and colleagues that they would return with something to justify the time away.

Taking trainees out of their normal environment gave them time to reflect on what they had learned. They were in classroom sessions all day, and then, in the evenings, worked on group work assignments to present the following day. This created a sense of common purpose and pride that would not have been possible with a day program or online format. For many participants, an online modality would also have been challenging due to unreliable internet connectivity.

The course demanded the full attention of trainees and required that they set aside their organizational status. They were instructed to "leave their professional hats at the door" and work with one another as equal collaborators in problem-based learning to improve PNG's health sector. This approach was essential to breaking down the siloed approach to management that impedes progress in the health system. For some of the senior clinicians used to being in authority, this was a challenging experience, and was often described by them as humbling. It not only required those used to being the ones talking to stay quiet and listen, but also empowered those who generally deferred to others in their workplace to find their voice and actively participate.

The course facilitators, both local and international, were all highly knowledgeable on their subjects as they applied to the local context. The theory and concepts were always directly tied to the trainees' own environment and professional challenges. Class discussions around real-world PNG examples enabled trainees to share their personal experiences. They were able to learn from others whom they would otherwise not have been in contact with due to isolation from peers in other provinces and agencies, as well as the communication siloes within their own organization, separating, for example, hospital clinical and corporate services.

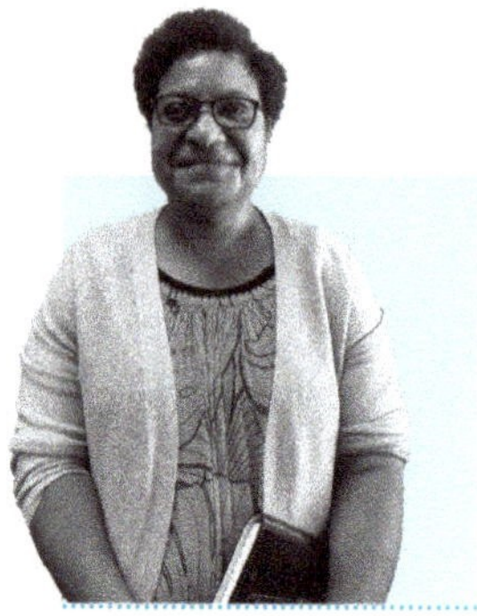

Martina Suve-Hohora

Executive Manager, Strategic Policy Division, National Department of Health

"This course got me to think of my objectives and purpose, to understand my place within the health sector, what I contribute. I am able to see beyond my scope of work to realize the broader vision of the sector and how I can contribute toward achieving that."

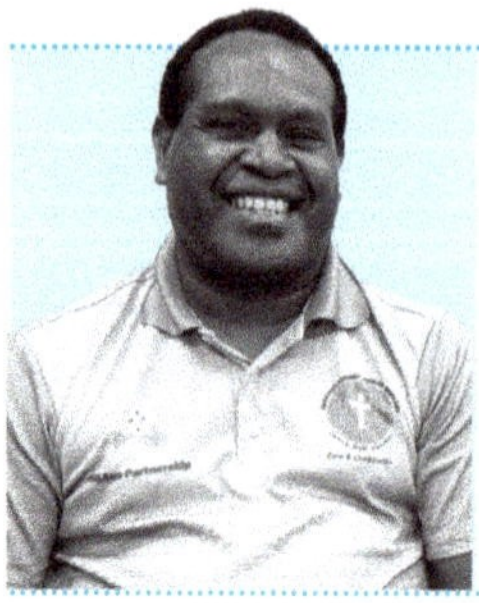

Graham Apian

Projects Director, Catholic Church Health Services

"From the very beginning, when we entered the room, the message was: you're one team. You're learning together to improve the health sector in PNG, and I think that really set the tone right throughout the training. Everyone could really cooperate well and learn from each other."

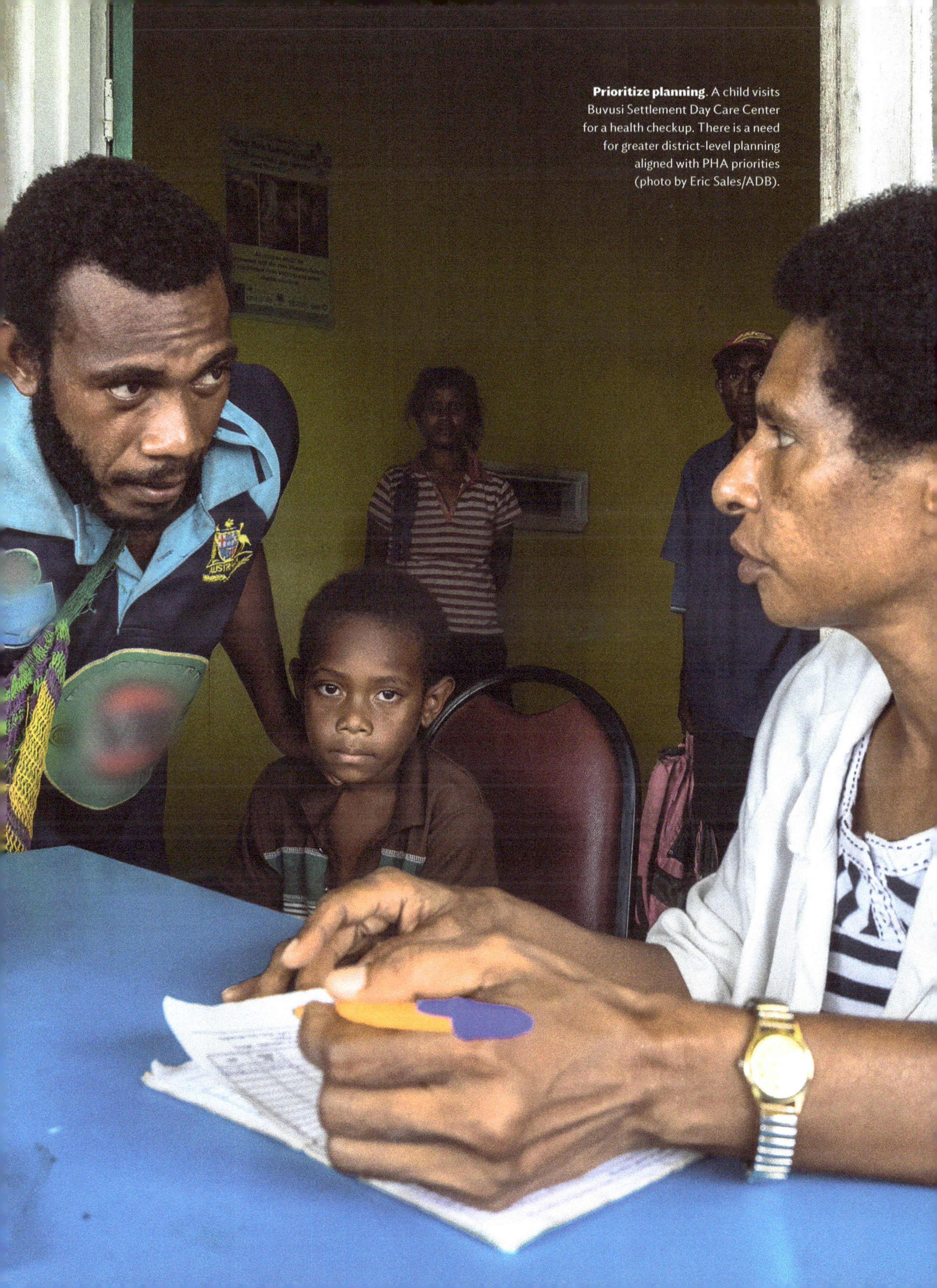

Prioritize planning. A child visits Buvusi Settlement Day Care Center for a health checkup. There is a need for greater district-level planning aligned with PHA priorities (photo by Eric Sales/ADB).

Insights and Inspiration from the Training

When interviewed about HELDP, both graduates and their supervisors were overwhelmingly positive about the impact of the training. They described how it had changed their way of working, including encouraging them to be more strategic, rational and analytical. They left the training with a new appreciation of what they could bring to their organizations and a greater understanding of their role in a team, and that of their colleagues in other departments.

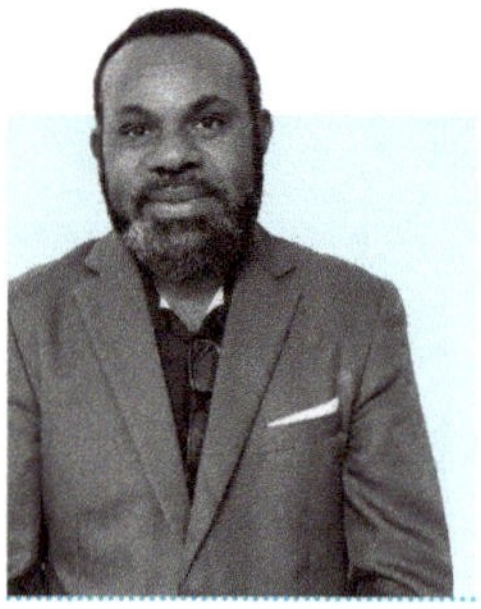

Dr Martin Daimen

Chief Executive Officer, Madang PHA

"Strategy, critical thinking, and analytical skills are key to any health executive leadership career. The course was tailored to those who already had some management experience, and mentoring them to become health leaders."

NEED FOR A MORE STRATEGIC MINDSET

Trainees realized that their ground-level focus on dealing with daily operations and exerting control to keep staff on track was not helpful in a leadership role. The course pushed trainees to think beyond their usual processes and develop a more visionary and strategic mindset, and to take a more expansive view of their purpose and contribution to the health sector. For those already engaged in policy and planning, the training reoriented their thinking to include the mechanics of implementation. An important part of the training process was gaining knowledge of themselves, their own strengths and shortcomings, and how to read other people's behavior.

One of the key insights from the training was the participants' tendency to favor existing ways of working, as if this somehow protected an organization's legacy. The training helped participants understand that they would need to re-strategize if they wanted to see change. For example, the structure of the health care workforce uses a model that was created in the 1970s and is highly hospital-centric. However, this is no longer fit for purpose in a country with a much larger population, changing disease patterns, and a growing need for primary health care and health promotion, often in remote, hard-to-reach communities.

Course participants grew in confidence as advocates for the health sector within the political system, and saw the need to engage with politics to ensure the sector gets the priority status it deserves. They developed a sense of common purpose across PHAs and other health organizations, despite the PHAs being at different stages of maturity.

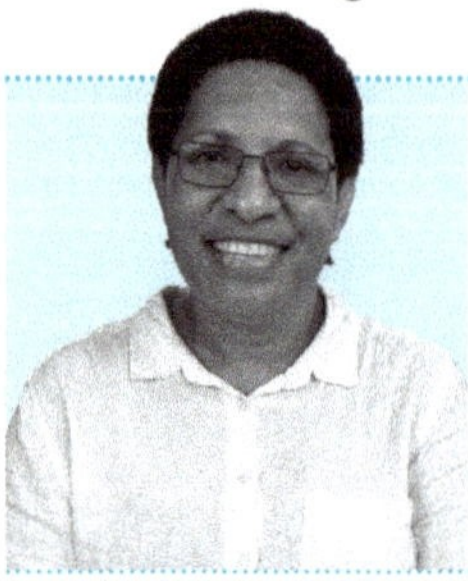

Gabriella Ak

Acting Pathology Services Coordinator, Port Moresby General Hospital

"I was empowered to rethink the way instead of just accepting the status quo. Before, I thought we had to protect that legacy, which didn't allow for a different way of thinking. The course helped me to realize we have to re-strategize if we want to see change."

LEADERS AS THE BRIDGE FROM POLICY TO ACTION

As senior executives in the health system, trainees were aware of the national policies and strategies affecting the health system, including the PNG National Health Plan and the National Health Service Standards, as well as more specific plans, for example, for malaria control. However, for clinicians on the ground, these often seemed detached from their day-to-day work. The course defined their role as leaders in influencing their team to be more strategic, and ensure that the national vision for health care is cascaded down through the health system, from province to district and communities. In this way, staff at all levels of the health system can develop a sense of contributing to a greater goal.

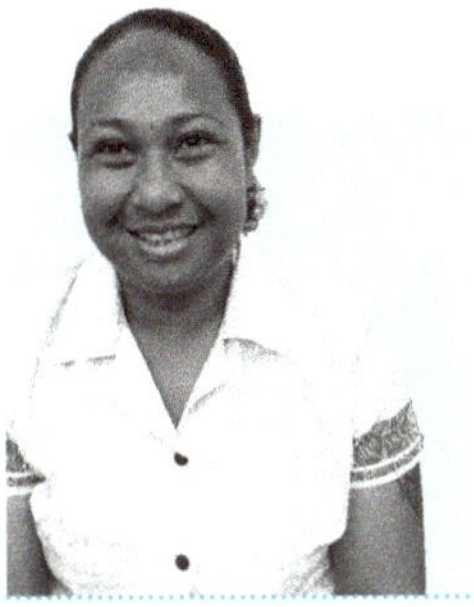

Vellgie Ava

Manager, Program Quality and Case Management, Rotarians Against Malaria

"During this course, I realized I had to get our national strategic plans and make them known to my team, so now they know what we have to achieve, what we're working toward."

EVERYONE CAN TEACH ... AND LEARN

Bringing together a diverse range of people created rich opportunities to develop a shared understanding and devise common pathways to resolving issues and crises in their respective work environments. It also trained them in incorporating the perspectives of others into a wider group.

As well as breaking down barriers between different health sector professions, the training also forged new connections across the government, PHA, private and NGO sectors. Trainees learned about the unique challenges facing colleagues in other organizations and departments, and were exposed to diverse ways of analyzing and solving problems.

Training leaders together from across the range of health care professions, rather than, for example, running training for physicians or nurses alone, gave participants a common understanding that would not have been reached if they had been trained according to their profession. For trainees whose colleagues also attended, that shared language could then be brought into senior executive management meetings. This reduced time spent trying to convince colleagues and created more time to achieve set goals.

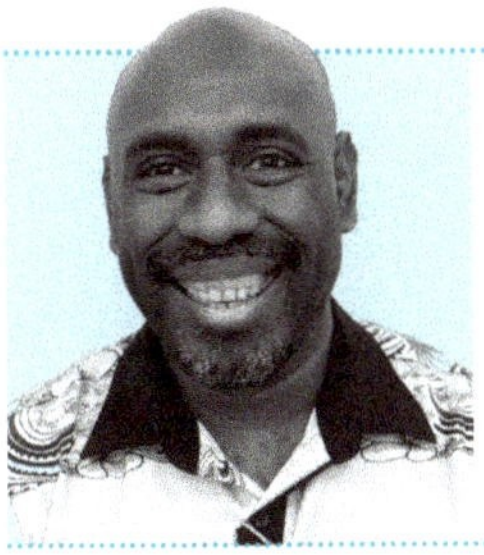

Daniel Kanasa

General Surgeon, Port Moresby General Hospital

"Sitting with [members of] different professions in the health space, there was a lot of diversity in how to analyze and deal with matters, and that was an eye-opener for me as a doctor."

LEADERSHIP, MANAGEMENT, AND GOVERNANCE IN THE MELANESIAN CONTEXT

The course acknowledges that health system leaders are often caught between Melanesian and Western values. Achieving results for a PHA in this context requires the leaders to strike a balance between often conflicting cultures. This can be at a philosophical level— such as favoring communitarianism over individualism, and hierarchy over equality—but also on a practical level, such as tolerance of lateness versus punctuality, and staff's expectation of time off being granted for family obligations versus observing strict boundaries between work and personal time.

The training program took an approach that recognized and respected Melanesian cultural values and explored how to capitalize on health standards improvement through collectivism, respect, and community involvement, particularly in rural areas. Modules on leadership, for example, promoted inclusive decision-making and ethical leadership consistent with local norms.

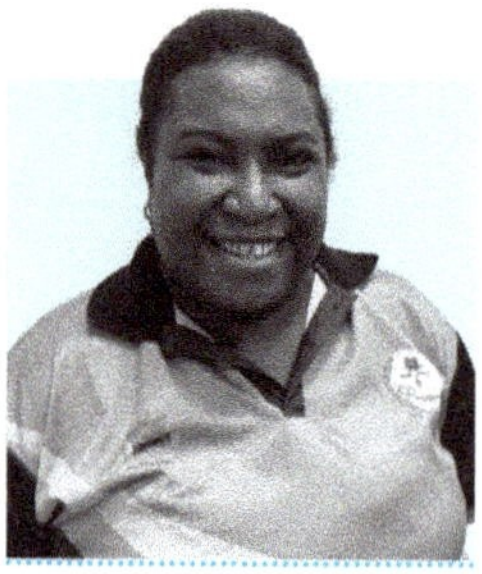

Regina Tomtai

Rural Outreach Officer, Madang PHA

“The course empowered me, giving me confidence that I can do better, and also to encourage young women, being a role model to my team, especially other nurses.”

Gender dimension of leadership

Women accounted for about one-third of the trainees. For many women that had risen to senior positions, lack of confidence was not an issue, but in a culture that favors deference to men, they often hesitated to voice their opinions. The course helped women overcome this barrier and exert their influence over leadership and management decisions, and recognize the importance of networking and self-promotion. The course explicitly encouraged those who were shy to overcome their reticence, giving them the confidence to speak out, and a belief that their voices counted.

Gender norms were just one aspect of Melanesian culture that came up in the training. Through intensive group work built around typical scenarios encountered in their work, trainees developed skills in navigating the two cultures. It also sensitized them to the need to deftly navigate cultural differences between different parts of the country, and even from one community to another.

OVERSEAS STUDY TOUR

Although only accounting for 10 days of the 9-week training period, the overseas study tour had an outsized impact on the trainees. It took the theoretical concepts learned in the classes and demonstrated how they were being applied on a daily basis in organizational environments (Figure 6). Faculty from UPNG accompanied the participants on the tours, which was also beneficial to them, as they gained exposure they could then use in future teaching activities. Meetings with senior staff at the host organizations reinforced the importance of strong and visionary leadership.

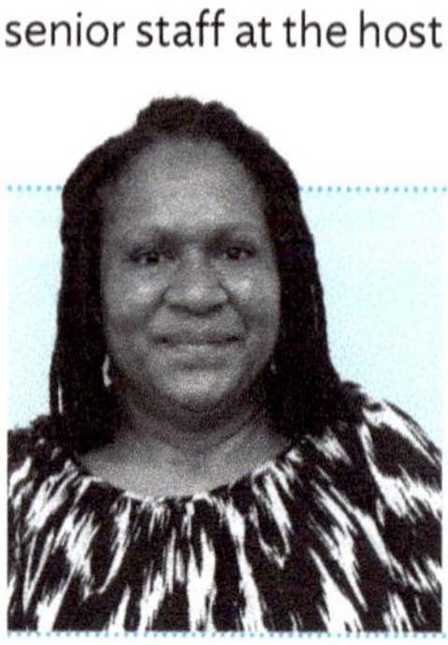

Theresia Mangi

General Services Manager, Port Moresby General Hospital

“The overseas study tour was the experience of a lifetime, meeting health workers in different hospitals and settings, and seeing different ways to manage a health system.”

Figure 6: Study Tour Destinations

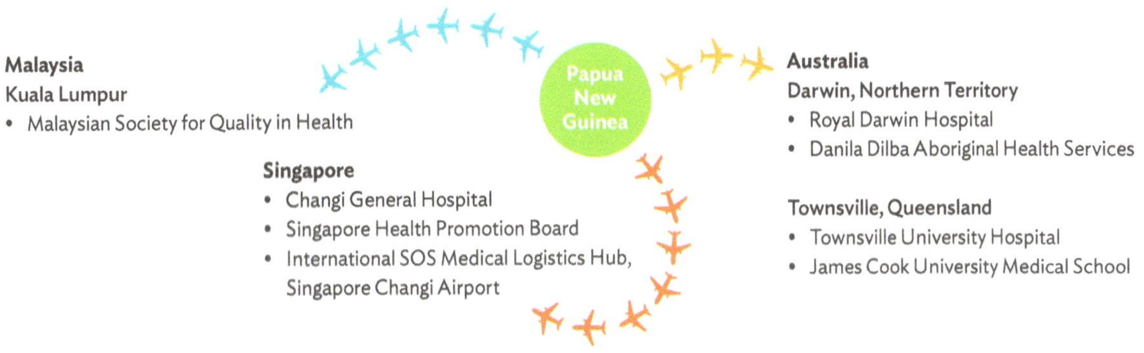
Malaysia
Kuala Lumpur
• Malaysian Society for Quality in Health
Papua New Guinea
Singapore
• Changi General Hospital
• Singapore Health Promotion Board
• International SOS Medical Logistics Hub, Singapore Changi Airport
Australia
Darwin, Northern Territory
• Royal Darwin Hospital
• Danila Dilba Aboriginal Health Services
Townsville, Queensland
• Townsville University Hospital
• James Cook University Medical School

Better ways of working

At Townsville University Hospital in Queensland, Australia, trainees observed how the leadership team routinely referred to a live dashboard to follow hospital operations, such as bed occupancy and clinical activities. This illustrated how routine, sex-disaggregated data collection fed into decision-making, such as for procurement and planning. The trainees not only saw technology in action, but also the way management operated. For example, when presenting their priorities and objectives, management also detailed the implementation process needed to achieve their objectives. The trainees also noted aspects of the work culture that their host organizations took for granted, including teamwork, patient-focused care, cleanliness, and punctuality. These experiences inspired the trainees to think differently about their own practices.

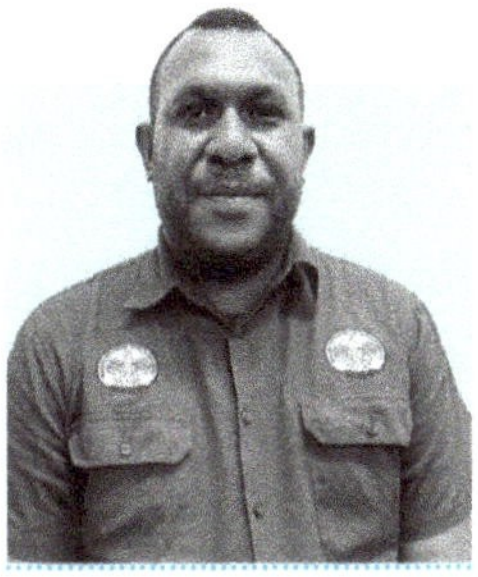

Dr Juith Gawi

Director, Curative Health Services, Madang PHA

"The overseas exposure was mind-blowing. This really changed the way I saw things from a management point of view."

The visits to the Malaysian Society for Quality in Health in Kuala Lumpur, showed how standards and accreditation are key to connecting overarching health system goals with clinical governance implementation and structures, through clearly defined and measurable processes and outcomes, leading to best patient care practices, and safe, effective, and sustainable health care services delivery. The Malaysian experience also showed how standards and accreditation can be raised over time, rather than setting unrealistic goals at the outset, which can then seem impossible to reach.

Similarly, the Singapore Health Promotion Board visit showcased what can be achieved when health promotion is treated as a core component of the health system rather than as an optional add-on that bears no relation to the business of a hospital. It also reinforced the need for the health sector to collaborate with other stakeholders to make the changes necessary for population health, such as tobacco control, or limiting sugar use in processed foods.

Progress is on a continuum

One of the intentions of the overseas study tour was to show trainees that they are on a journey of progress, and that others who are ahead of them were at their stage in the past, and reached their goals step by step. They found that there were not only differences, but also similarities. In Northern Australia, they saw how services for remote Aboriginal communities were being made more accessible through the upskilling of rural health workers in ways that could be adapted to rural PNG. The trainees heard firsthand from service providers that it was possible to improve service offerings through better management even within budgetary constraints.

Technology

One aspect of the overseas settings that really stood out for trainees was technology use. For example, they observed how automated pathology services in Singapore increased the throughput capacity of a laboratory and enabled clinicians to promptly access patient test results via their mobile phones. They saw how artificial intelligence and robotics were being used to perform basic tasks, such as patient food delivery, to free up nurses' for more clinical care. Some of these automated activities are aspirational even in developed country settings, but they all found purchase with the trainees, inspiring them to embrace automation rather than see it as a challenge to the workforce in PNG's more manual-focused system.

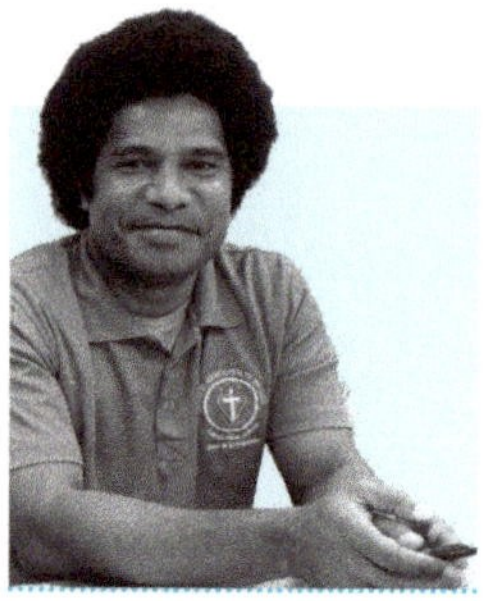

Athanasius Kari

Director of Rural Health Development, Catholic Church Health Services

"

[The study tour] put into practice all the theory we were learning throughout the course, especially when we had sessions that talked about technology, improving the health space in a digital way."

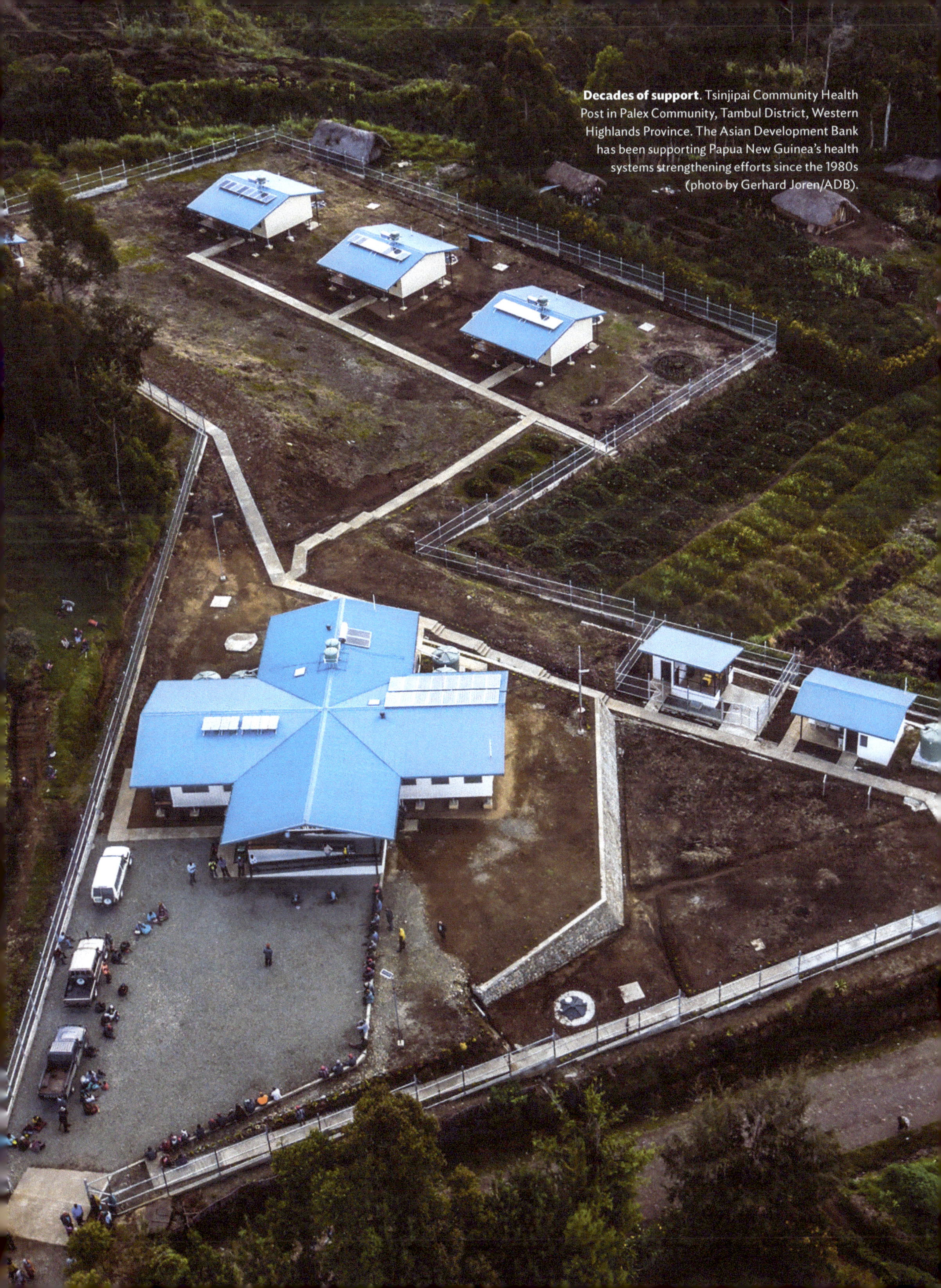

Decades of support. Tsinjipai Community Health Post in Palex Community, Tambul District, Western Highlands Province. The Asian Development Bank has been supporting Papua New Guinea's health systems strengthening efforts since the 1980s (photo by Gerhard Joren/ADB).

Beyond Theory to Practice: What Changed After the Training

Graduates, their managers, and other stakeholders in the program have observed the results of the training. The program has led to visibly improved leadership confidence, decision-making, and organizational performance. At an institutional level, there is evidence of better coordination within PHAs and stronger alignment with national health strategies (Figure 7).

When they returned to their workplaces, graduates reported being more able to incorporate other people's perspectives, ask questions and listen more. They became more focused on solutions instead of bemoaning the status quo. Their people-management skills had improved, especially in conflict resolution and discipline. They had a stronger sense of the importance of data for evaluation and results monitoring.

Those who were not already in senior leadership positions realized that there were future career pathways for them in health sector leadership. Several graduates have moved into more senior positions. Those who have been promoted attribute their success to the training they received. It gave them the confidence to pursue promotion and helped them stand out and excel in interviews. Several others are in the process of applying for promotion.

Priya Balusubramaniam
HELDP facilitator

"There's a marked difference after the course in the people I've worked with for many years. They're a lot more responsive, and they can talk at a higher level, look at the bigger picture, and they can talk about longer-term strategy."

Figure 7: What Changed After the Leadership Training

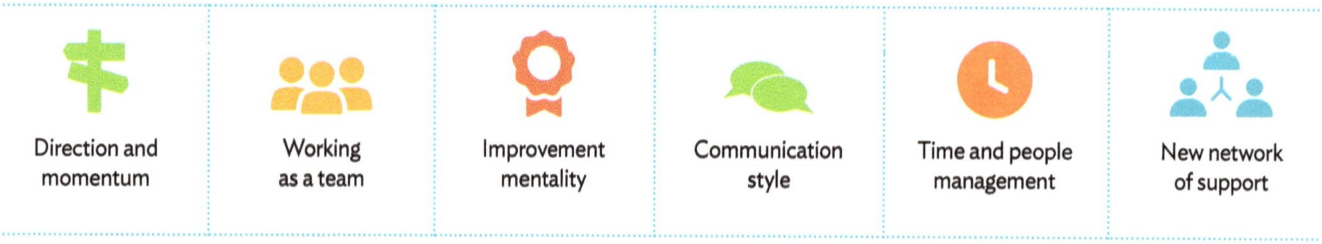

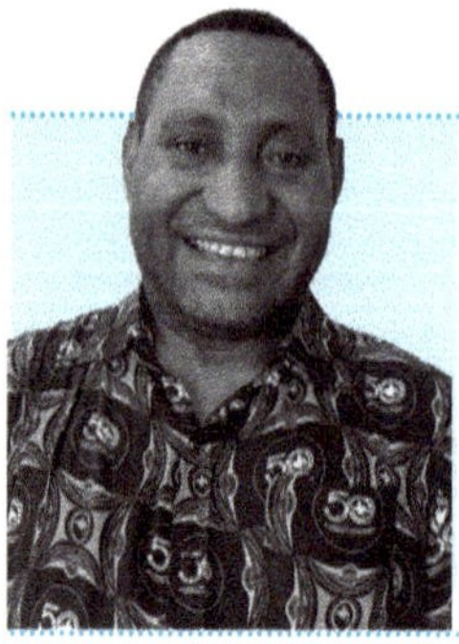

Scotty Kandelyo
Executive Clinical Standards Manager, National Department of Health

"HELDP is contextualized to our health system and helped us to see, from a strategic perspective, how we can best manage the system."

DIRECTION AND MOMENTUM

In Western Highlands PHA, where six members of the senior executive management team completed the HELDP training, the change was palpable, according to the PHA's chief executive, Jane Holden. The PHA has outperformed all others in the country for the past two years, after a period of concerted effort to reorganize and improve service delivery.

The chief executive credits HELDP with training her staff in the skills they needed to coalesce as a team around shared goals, and navigate the PHA's many competing priorities, based on evidence and rational decision-making. The training enabled the PHA to build momentum in its reforms. "We need to manage competing priorities and, if we haven't got leaders—who understand decision-making processes, who can prioritize, who can look at returns on investment, who can objectively consider economic returns on investment and all these things—we are never going to move forward," Holden said.

Similarly, in Madang PHA—the worst-performing in the country in 2024—the chief executive appointed in September 2025 is a HELDP graduate, and is using what he learned to identify and analyze problems, and galvanize his senior management team as he embarks on changing the PHA's model of care and transforming service delivery.

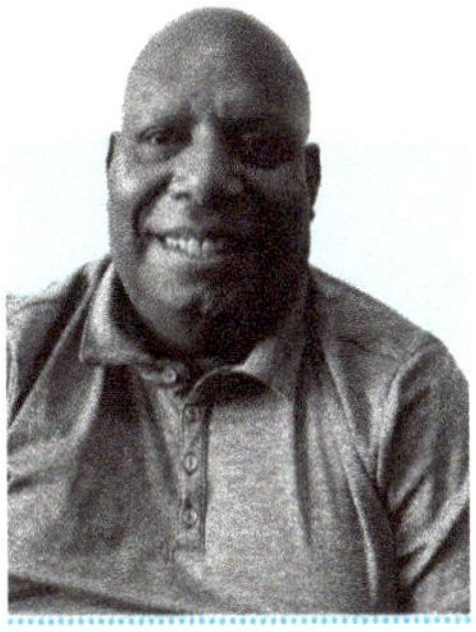

Dannax Kupamo

Director for Public Health, Western Highlands PHA

"After coming back from the training, there was total shift, and then we saw our indicators improve for two consecutive years, to become the top-performing PHA. Now we work in unison, and there's communication flow across all the directorates, and I think we are now one team."

WORKING AS A TEAM

Both the clinical staff and the corporate and support services staff who graduated from HELDP have changed their view of colleagues outside their own profession. Each group now has a greater appreciation of the work of the other, and a new recognition that they are all on the same team playing crucial roles in patient care, even when they are not patient facing. Communication between clinical and corporate services improved when executive level staff had been trained through HELDP.

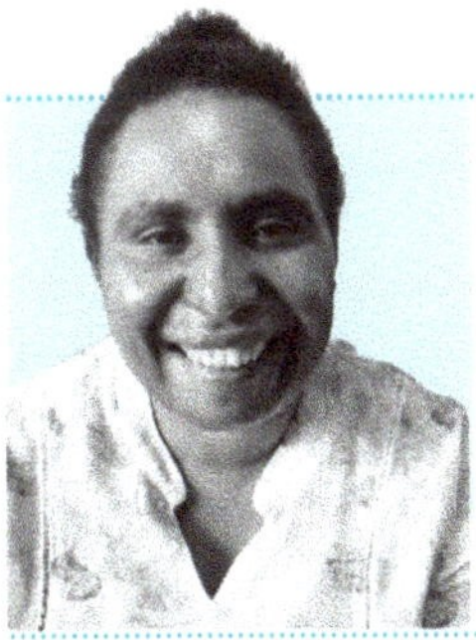

Jokeybeth Damieng

Deputy Director, Finance and Administration, Western Highlands PHA

"Previously, the clinicians saw us in corporate as a separate team but, after the training, I'm seeing that things are beginning to change. The program has really had an impact on how people think and approach others."

IMPROVEMENT MENTALITY

Graduates described a change in their mentality, with a greater tendency to identify what could be done better with existing resources, and ways to be effective and efficient, and then save time. There is a growing culture of evidence-based advocacy and decision-making. Although the hospital systems observed by the trainees on the study tour were better resourced and more advanced in data collection, their processes can be replicated in the PNG context. For example, one medical services director adopted the clinical governance processes he had seen in Australia and reformed the data flow on hospital deaths. This led to improvements in patient safety and hospital accountability, and fostered an improvement culture among his staff. Graduates have become more motivated to take the initiative and make changes.

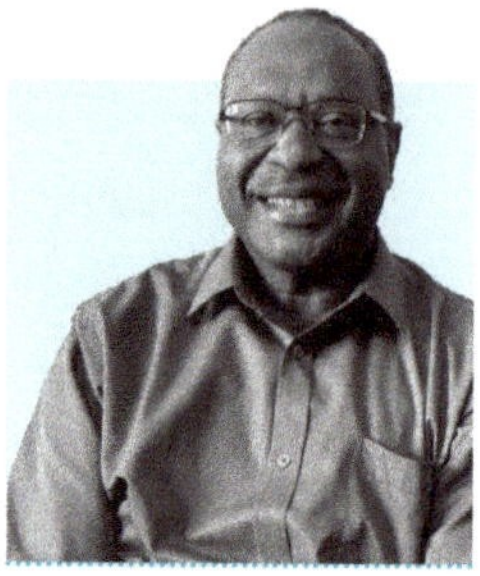

Jonah Kurubi

Deputy Director, Medical Services, Western Highlands PHA

"After returning from the study tour at Townsville University Hospital in Australia, I implemented key clinical governance practices to strengthen quality improvement, accountability, and patient safety programs within our hospital."

COMMUNICATION STYLE

Another important element of the training was communication. Graduates described being better equipped to speak up and lead their teams. This was particularly so for some of the female participants. They returned to their workplaces resolved to advocate for themselves and their ideas, and to be role models for women in more junior positions. While medical and nursing training equips clinicians for communication in the context of individual patient care, this is not helpful when they become managers and need to have the confidence to speak in public. Extroverts were sensitized to the need to pay attention to quieter team members, draw them into the conversation, and listen more actively, and have brought this change into their senior executive, management and staff meetings.

Communication skills are also helping with discipline and motivation. One senior hospital manager found that she had shifted from seeing her role as hiring and firing people, to helping her staff improve, retaining good employees and supporting them to work better. Another NDOH executive changed her management style away from criticism to encouragement to perform better, and found it was more effective in motivating people to change.

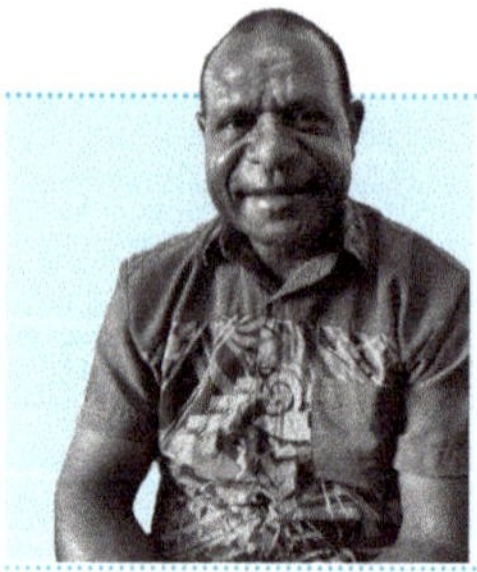

Madison Dat

Deputy Director, Curative Health Services, Western Highlands PHA

"As a clinician, you are trained to talk to an individual patient, but then, when you need to talk to a group of people, that's a bit of a challenge. The training gave us that confidence to communicate, get people to engage, and lead them together as a team."

TIME AND PEOPLE MANAGEMENT

Graduates reported making changes to how they manage issues that they now perceive as hampering productivity, such as poor time management and lack of punctuality. Having seen how the Malaysian health system manages standards and accreditation, two of the graduates began to question how the PNG National Health Service Standards are being met in their hospital. As the first step toward improvement, they began with a survey to rate themselves and their senior colleagues.

People management—including knowledge of self—was a key component of the HELDP curriculum, and participants learned the skills to help them navigate the different perspectives of others. One of the PNG-specific challenges the graduates have to navigate is the extent to which family and community obligations need to be balanced against work roles. One graduate is working to redress the balance in favor of work by running professional development courses and staff retention programs to instill the same disciplined and committed mindset that she herself gained from the HELDP training.

NEW NETWORK OF SUPPORT

Each cohort of graduates formed social media groups, and these have remained active as a source of news sharing, mutual support, advice and discussion. These groups enable people to stay connected, not only to their professional peers in other provinces, but also to colleagues from other professions in the health system that they would not ordinarily have met.

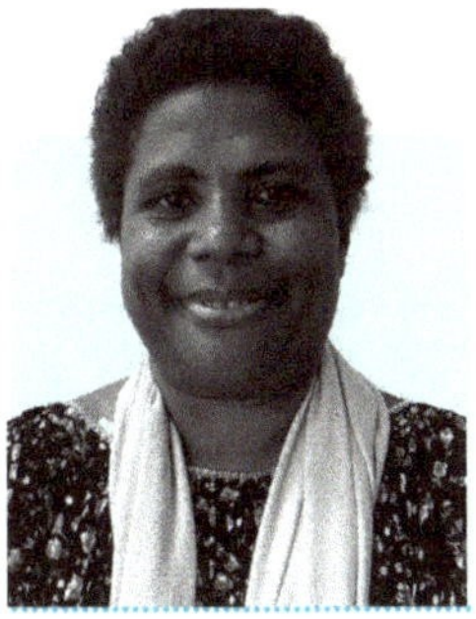

Lillian Urae

Human Resources Manager, Western Highlands PHA

"I've changed a lot in terms of being able to consider what other people think and feel, and in terms of understanding the organization and what it requires of me."

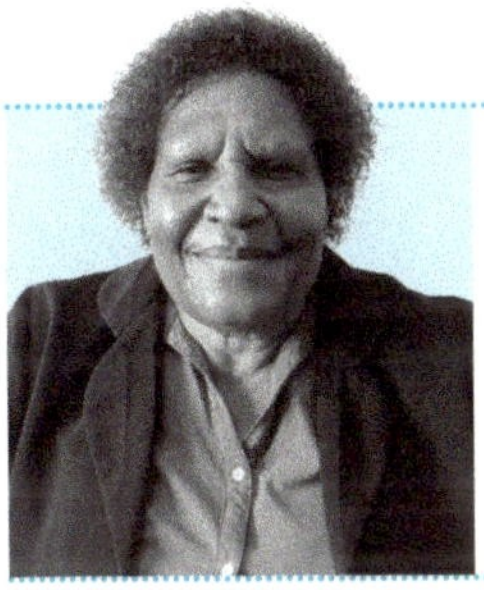

Serah Dot

Hospital Manager, Mount Hagen General Hospital

"In Malaysia, the way they talked about standards and accreditation really challenged me. Afterwards, we did a survey to look at whether we were practicing within the National Health Service Standards in our hospital and practicing to the standards we've seen overseas."

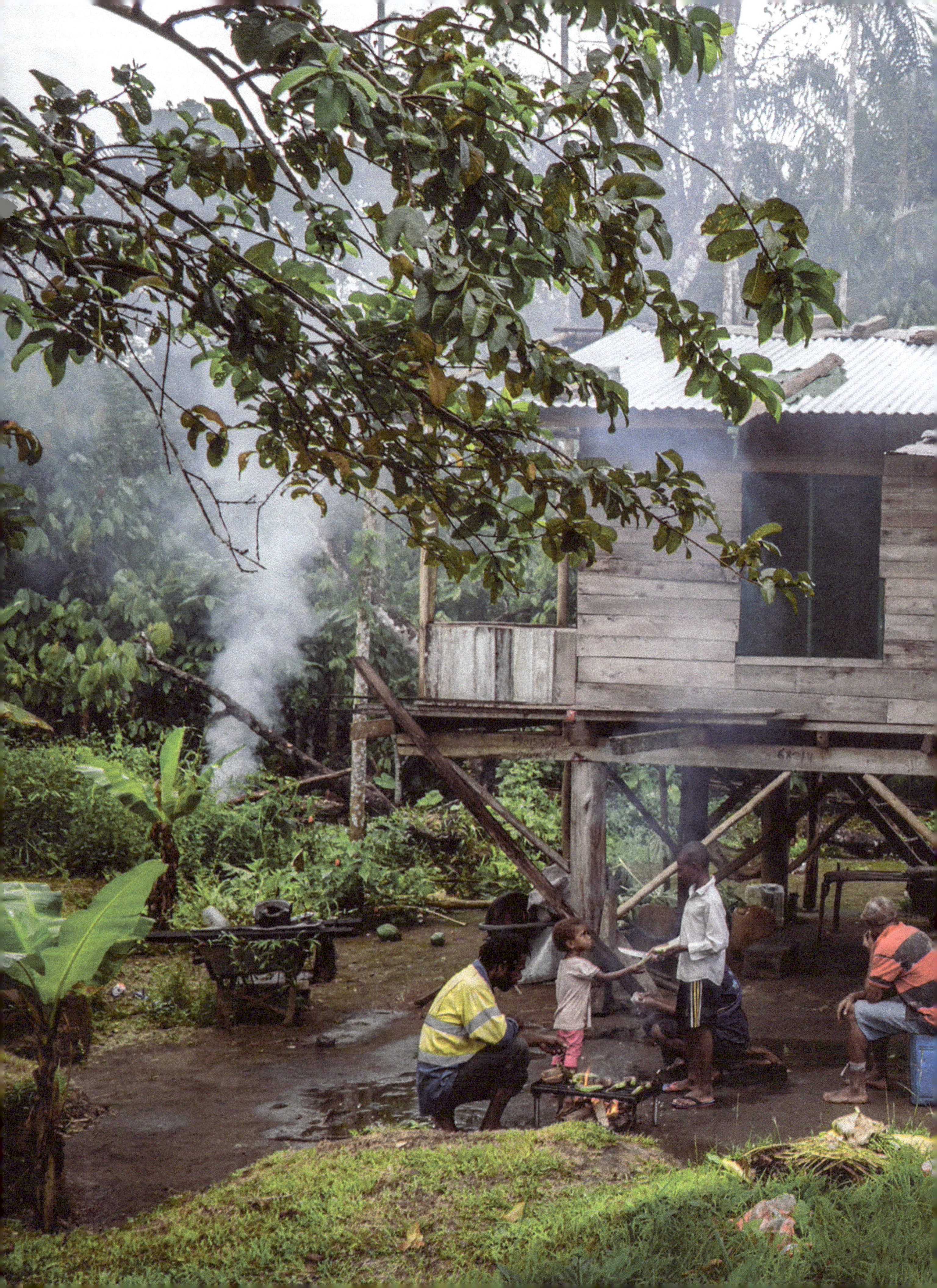

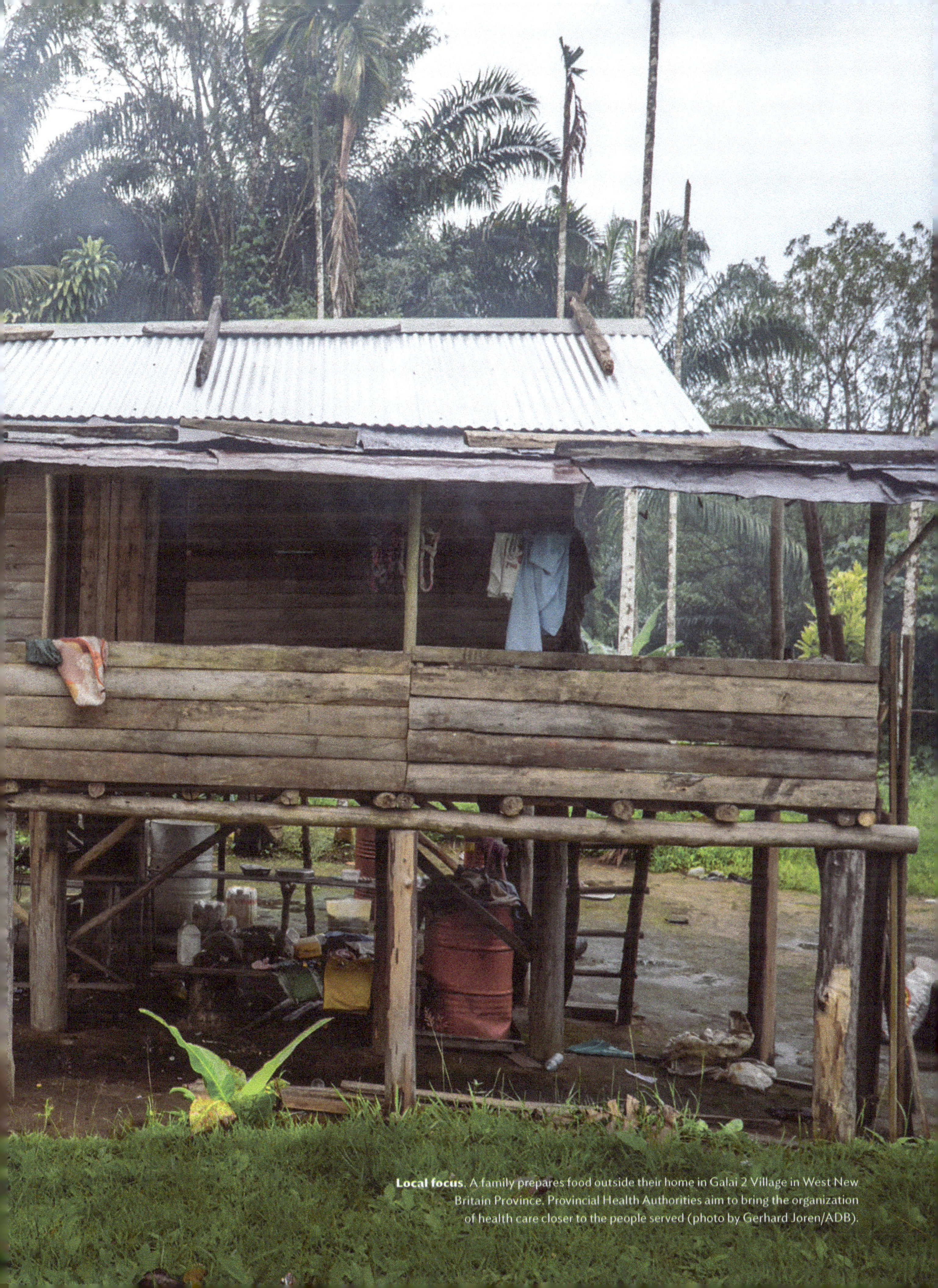

Local focus. A family prepares food outside their home in Galai 2 Village in West New Britain Province. Provincial Health Authorities aim to bring the organization of health care closer to the people served (photo by Gerhard Joren/ADB).

Graduate Projects

All graduates were required to work on a final project that would bring about change in their work setting. Several initiated service delivery improvement projects, improved data use in planning, and enhanced team management and communication in their provinces. Below are some examples of projects.

All graduates were required to work on a final project that would bring about change in their work setting.

HEALTH DATA COLLECTION

For Sally Laka, Monitoring and Evaluations Coordinator at Catholic Church Health Services (CCHS), data collection lies at the heart of her work. The quality of information received from health facilities determines how effectively CCHS can monitor progress, measure outcomes, and make evidence-based decisions. Incomplete, delayed, or inaccurate data limits the ability to identify gaps and support improvements in service delivery.

Working in a data-driven environment, Laka often faced the challenge of reviewing long and detailed reports. She wanted a more creative way to communicate key ideas that would be easier for others to understand and remember. Inspired by how short television commercials quickly capture attention and deliver strong messages, she decided to use a similar approach for her final project.

Laka produced a short video, *The Significance of Health Data: Your Role Matters*, aimed at raising awareness among health workers about the value of quality data and their role in collecting and managing it.[14] The video tells the story of how the CCHS data systems evolved, from paper logbooks to digital repositories, showing how reliable data collection supports dashboard generation, trend analysis, and informed planning. Ultimately, it demonstrates that quality data is more than just numbers; it is the foundation for improving health services and advocating for better resource allocation.

CLINICAL WASTE MANAGEMENT

HELDP graduate Gabriella Ak is Acting Pathology Services Coordinator at Port Moresby General Hospital. As chair of its infection prevention control committee, she saw gaps in the waste management system, particularly in how clinical waste was stored prior to collection. As the hospital has ambitions to become a tertiary referral research hospital, Ak knew that standards for clinical waste management had to be improved.

On returning to the hospital after the HELDP training, she designed a new waste management flow, from the patient's bed to final incineration, including improvements to the waste storage facility. She successfully advocated for hospital funding, and the facility has been in operation since September 2025. Clinical waste is now centrally collected and sealed in an air-conditioned storage space. The process enables collection trucks to empty the storage containers and return them in a safe and hygienic way.

---

[14] Catholic Church Health Services. The Significance of Health Data: Your Role Matters.

ASSETS REGISTRY

Tony Basse, Acting Coordinator for District Health Services at Eastern Highlands PHA, was aware that information about the authority's physical assets was scattered across different places, and there was no way to keep track of them. This data is essential for service planning. For his final project, Basse, who has a passion for database systems and was looking for an opportunity to make a meaningful contribution to his PHA, set about designing an assets registry. He envisioned a user-friendly, sustainable, centralized and cloud-based registry that could be managed locally by the PHA at very minimal cost. He also hoped that this work would pave the way for other PHAs to do the same.

The assets registry would provide a clear overview of all the authority's physical assets, making it easier to monitor their status and location, and track their life cycle.

The registry would provide a clear overview of all assets, making it easier to monitor their status and location, and track their life cycle. This in turn would facilitate accurate asset valuation, which is needed for financial reporting, and to meet legal and regulatory requirements. It would also improve operational efficiency through better identification of underutilized or redundant assets, and planning for future asset needs and investments based on data-driven measurement of return on investment. By improving loss prevention and supporting insurance claims, it would help manage the PHA's risk, and would support its auditing process and transparency. When assets reached the end of their useful life, the digital assets registry would also facilitate their disposal and recycling in an environmentally responsible way.

Basse's project convened a team to develop the software for an assets registry database that would be compatible for use on the existing PHA local area network. The software has been developed and, pending senior executive management endorsement for use, will centralize the procurement and distribution system within the PHA. The next step for Basse, who in his current role is assisting the standards division of Eastern Highlands PHA, is to develop other database systems that will be cost-effective, sustainable and user-friendly.

WELLNESS CENTERS

As well as looking after other people, health care workers also need to pay attention to their own well-being. Organizations with a culture that shows they care about their employees' health are more likely to enjoy strong employee engagement and higher productivity. With this in mind, and applying what he had learned in the training about meeting unmet needs, Jonah Kurubi, Deputy Director of Medical Services, Western Highlands PHA, was thinking about how to improve the health profile of the PHA's staff.

Kurubi began by looking at the data: in 2022, well over 400 sick leave applications were registered, translating into more than 450 days of lost productivity. Acute upper respiratory tract infection was the common reason, but trauma-related injuries were also prevalent among nursing professionals. To try and reduce these numbers, Kurubi advocated for wellness clinics that would offer a comprehensive model of care, including disease prevention and health promotion messages, early screening, and detection of risk factors to be managed early and support staff with existing diseases that required hospital care.

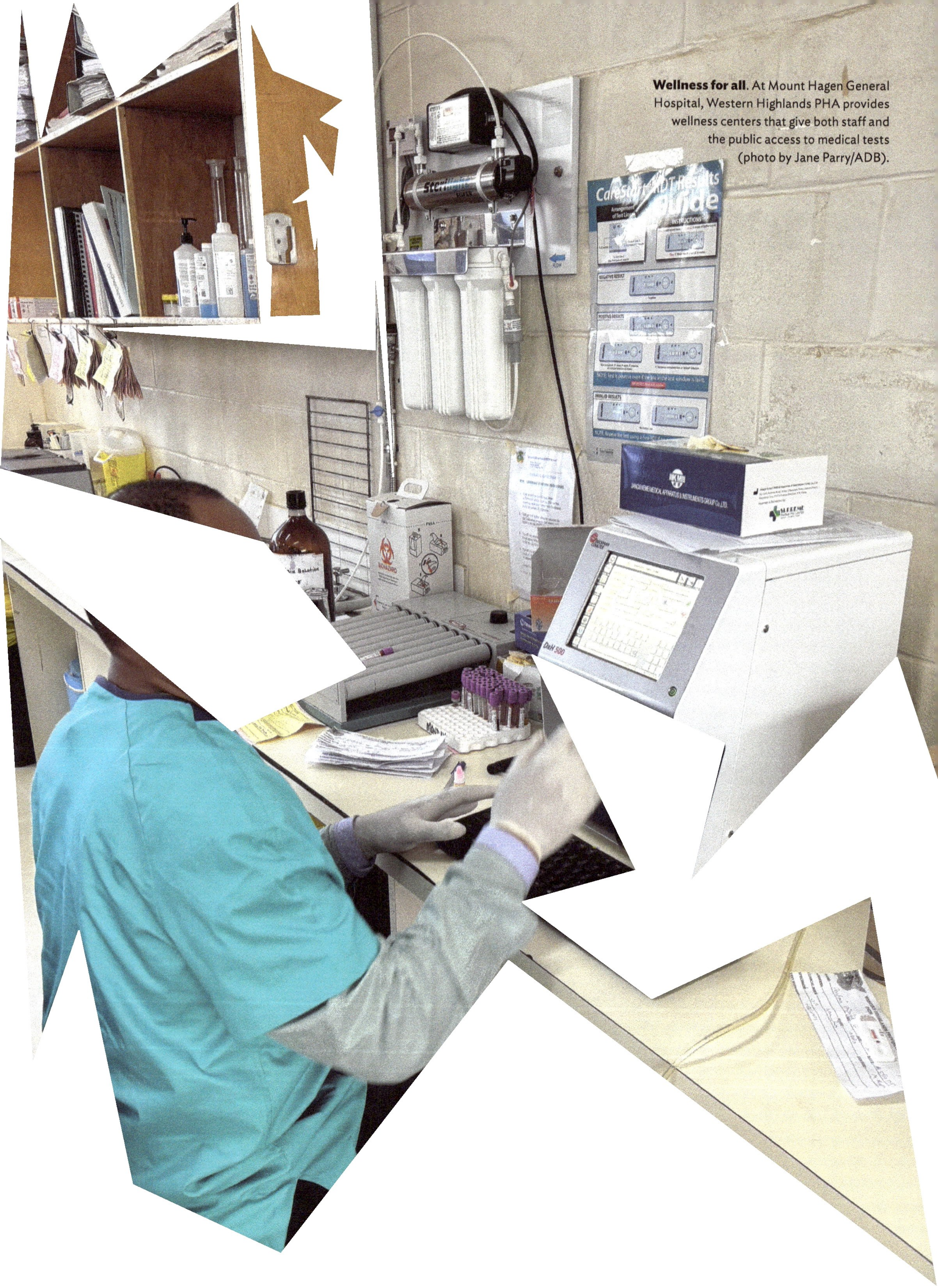

Wellness for all. At Mount Hagen General Hospital, Western Highlands PHA provides wellness centers that give both staff and the public access to medical tests (photo by Jane Parry/ADB).

The first wellness clinic began seeing staff in November that year. In the first 3 months of operation, more than 200 staff—about one-quarter of the PHA workforce—voluntarily participated, with women outnumbering men two to one (indicating that more advocacy is needed to encourage men to pay more attention to their health and well-being). Exhaustion and overweight were two common complaints cited by staff who attended the clinic. About one-fifth were unaware of their health issues until they registered in the wellness program; 4 staff were found to have diabetes and 27 had hypertension, and one-fifth of attendees were referred for specialist medical care.

The wellness clinics report data regularly to the PHA, strengthening surveillance, early intervention, and linkage to care for non-communicable disease.

Building on the success of the staff wellness clinic established at Mount Hagen General Hospital, Western Highlands PHA extended the initiative beyond staff well-being to include the general public. In 2024, the organization officially launched community wellness clinics across the province to promote non-communicable disease prevention and control. In 2024 and 2025, eight district health facilities became fully operational, providing routine wellness checks, lifestyle counseling, and chronic disease screening. These sites are now regularly reporting wellness clinic data to the PHA, strengthening surveillance, early intervention, and linkage to care for non-communicable disease across the Western Highlands.

Reflections and Recommendations

By the time HELDP's fourth cohort graduates, the program will have trained up to 150 health system leaders. Participants have built a robust knowledge base and their perspectives have shifted significantly during the program, with the experiences of each cohort informing adjustments to the next cycle of the training program. Their cumulative experience can also inform future iterations of the project.

REFLECTIONS

For the individual graduates, the course has proven to be highly impactful and, in some cases, transformational. An independent evaluation of the program found it to be highly relevant and effective, and demonstrating a high degree of satisfaction among participants.[15] The evaluation rated the course as efficient, and as having a satisfactory development impact. It also found that HELDP's defined outcomes were met. Participants improved their knowledge and returned to their workplaces motivated to implement what they had learned. The domestic capacity for such training has been increased.

However, the evaluation questioned the long-term sustainability of the program in its current form, due to the high cost. Moreover, the current time frame (the funding runs to the end of 2025) makes it difficult to allow for an appropriate transition period to a program, for example, delivered directly by one or both of the universities involved.

Cost of inaction

The cost of domestic and international travel, and taking clinicians and system managers away from their demanding roles for 2 weeks at a time, made the costs of the course high. However, graduates said that the course better equipped them to run their health system more efficiently, make better use of their existing resources, and support the aim of a healthier population, all of which have a financial benefit.

Varying degrees of support

On their return to their institutions, not every trainee found acceptance of their new ideas, and their enthusiasm for change faltered amid the unwillingness of others. Due to resistance or opposition from their chief executives, some graduates found they were not supported in their PHAs when they tried to implement the change management projects they had designed during the course. This was less common in settings where there was a supportive chief executive and a critical mass of HELDP graduates who could drive an agenda of strategic vision and change.

Clement Manineng
Director, Divine Word University Center for Health Research and Diagnostics, and Board Member, Madang PHA

"The impact of the training is very clear. In Madang PHA, there are three or four graduates serving in leadership roles. They're already putting those skills and knowledge to use, and so we are expecting some very positive results to come from that."

[15] Elich L. PNG HSSDP Monitoring & Evaluation, Health Executive Leadership Development Program Review Report, 2025.

Unintended consequences

The training has also had unintended consequences. One chief executive noted that the selection of candidates gave an impression of favoritism, which then had to be addressed and explained. Meanwhile, some organizations are seeing more staff turnover, as staff realize that they have more opportunities to get into leadership positions than they had previously, which could be a destabilizing influence. Some of those whose colleagues moved on as a result of their training saw this more positively, knowing that like-minded individuals could now be found in other organizations across the health system.

Systemic transformation needs more than leadership training

However important leadership training is, on its own it cannot solve what ails the PNG health system. There are capacity constraints across the whole spectrum of human resources for health. Medical services at all levels require expansion, maintenance or refurbishment. Resources will always be scarce, and health care must compete with other domains of government for funding. What resources are allotted to health need to be consistent and reliable to facilitate proper planning. Some of the current ways in which health services, leadership career paths, and health system governance are designed need reform to remove inherent dysfunctions and obstacles to progress. Strong, effective leaders are needed to address the many competing priorities of the health system, yet systemic transformation is a prerequisite to fostering that very leadership. While leadership training is a necessary condition, alone it is insufficient to achieve meaningful and sustained systemic change.

Luke Ambu
HELDP Coordinator, and Lecturer, Human Resources Management Division, School of Business & Public Policy, University of Papua New Guinea

“

The trainees' openness to new ideas and desire to improve health outcomes was inspiring. We sincerely hope that, when they want to implement these ideas and make things work, the PHAs and stakeholders will provide funding and resources to support them, not only in implementation but sustainability.”

RECOMMENDATIONS

Double the number of HELDP graduates

Although there is no proven approach to determine the critical mass of graduates needed within a single organization to transform its leadership, graduates have found that the impact of their individual training is synergous when they work together with fellow graduates.

The PHA boards and chief executives supportive of HELDP have seen the benefits and recognize the need for leadership transformation. Similarly, the CHS and CCHS leadership have seen the value of the training to their organizations as they deal with ever more complex health care delivery. Continuing to run HELDP for a further 3–5 years, either in its current or a similar form, could make a significant impact on the overarching strategic framework of the health system, and would enable the training of a greater number of younger and more ambitious managers.

Western Highlands PHA chief executive Jane Holden said she had 6 graduates out of 14 in her team, but needed a few more, preferably not all in the same place, and including some district managers.

Martin Daimen

Chief Executive Officer, Madang PHA

"I would like to have at least three graduates every year, because I need a pool of strategic leaders. This will create a very good team with the same mindset, and will allow for succession planning."

Provide bespoke training to PHA chief executives

The PHA chief executives were excluded from HELDP, and not all PHAs are functioning optimally. There is some induction training for PHA chief executives, but it is more focused on practical matters such a reporting requirements. A bespoke leadership training program for chief executives, pitched at a much more strategic level and run over a shorter time span (such as one 3-week period), could reinforce the impact of HELDP by equipping participants with alternatives to their current practices in, for example, resource distribution decision-making, and productivity and performance measurement.

Figure 8: Recommendations

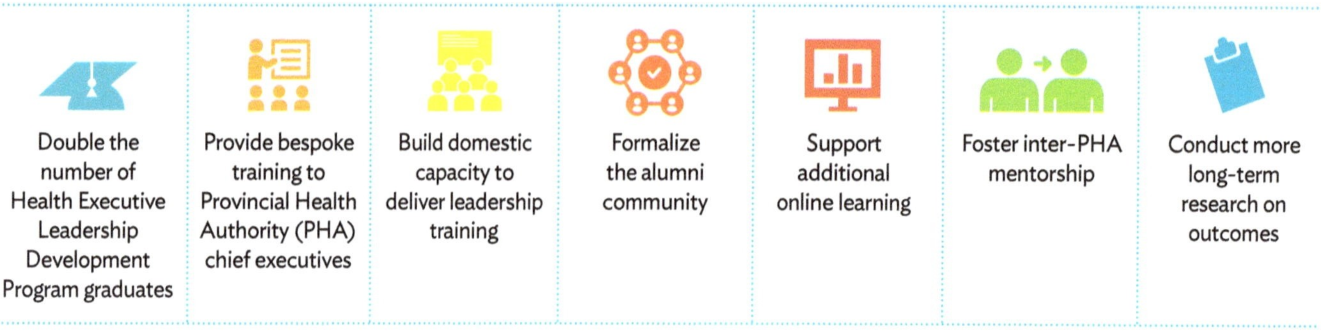

Build domestic capacity to deliver leadership training

Both UPNG and DWU are highly supportive of HELDP, and one way to ensure its sustainability would be to institutionalize the program within the two universities as a recognized postgraduate qualification, and a pathway to an in-house postgraduate diploma or master's degree. Such a pathway is impending. UPNG's School of Medicine & Health Sciences has developed a Master of Health Services Management degree curriculum, designed in partnership with UPNG's School of Business & Public Policy, and the HSSDP. The main target beneficiaries are the PHAs, with students drawn from the pool of health executives who hold managerial or supervisory positions. The program is earmarked to start in 2026, subject to university senate approval.

The main target beneficiaries are the PHAs, with students drawn from the pool of health executives who hold managerial or supervisory positions.

Continuing HELDP or running a similar program with a cost-sharing model between the NDOH and external assistance would buy time to transition to full domestic ownership and funding of the program. Domestic ownership of the program costs is important, not least because it galvanizes participants to work on truly transformative final projects that will be implemented within their organization.

Formalize the alumni community

Each cohort of graduates formed a social media group, and the chats continue to be active, as a forum to request help and advice, share news of achievements and promotions, and network. However, there is no mechanism for different cohorts to connect with each other. A graduate-led alumni alliance would facilitate more communication and the formation of a community of practice. Support for periodic events that bring graduates together would create opportunities for peer learning, such as through topic-specific online webinars. A "women in health" alumni network could help build and provide support to a pipeline of aspirant women leaders.

An in-person symposium would give graduates the opportunity to share the changes that they have made, enabling others to learn from their experience of policy change and system transformation. An alumni body would also encourage graduates to support the anticipated formation of the PNG chapter of the Australasian College of Health Service Management.

Support additional online learning

While the face-to-face, intensive and residential modality, combined with overseas exposure, is unique and highly effective, this training could be augmented with online programming if trainees were supported to access better online connectivity. This also dovetails with the international networking and continuing professional development opportunities that membership of the Australasian College of Health Service Management confers.

Foster inter-PHA mentorship

In time, study tours could also include visits to PHAs that are successfully transforming their health systems and service delivery, and there is also scope for ongoing inter-PHA support and mentorship. This could be in the form of a rotational program, for example, with graduates coming in to understudy chief executives around the country. Another potential modality is for senior executive managers to be released for several weeks a year, for placement in either high-performing or low-performing PHAs. This could evolve into a system of peer survey and accreditation, and enable structured, ongoing knowledge sharing on improvement.

Another potential modality is for senior executive managers to be released for several weeks a year, for placement in either high-performing or low-performing PHAs.

Conduct more long-term research on outcomes

The earliest cohort of graduates completed the course in March 2024. More time is needed to research and evaluate the extent to which the training has benefited and empowered them to bring about meaningful change. The required research includes both qualitative measurement of the long-term impact on PHA performance and health metrics, as well as qualitative research to understand why and how the graduates continue to take their executive training into their professional practice.

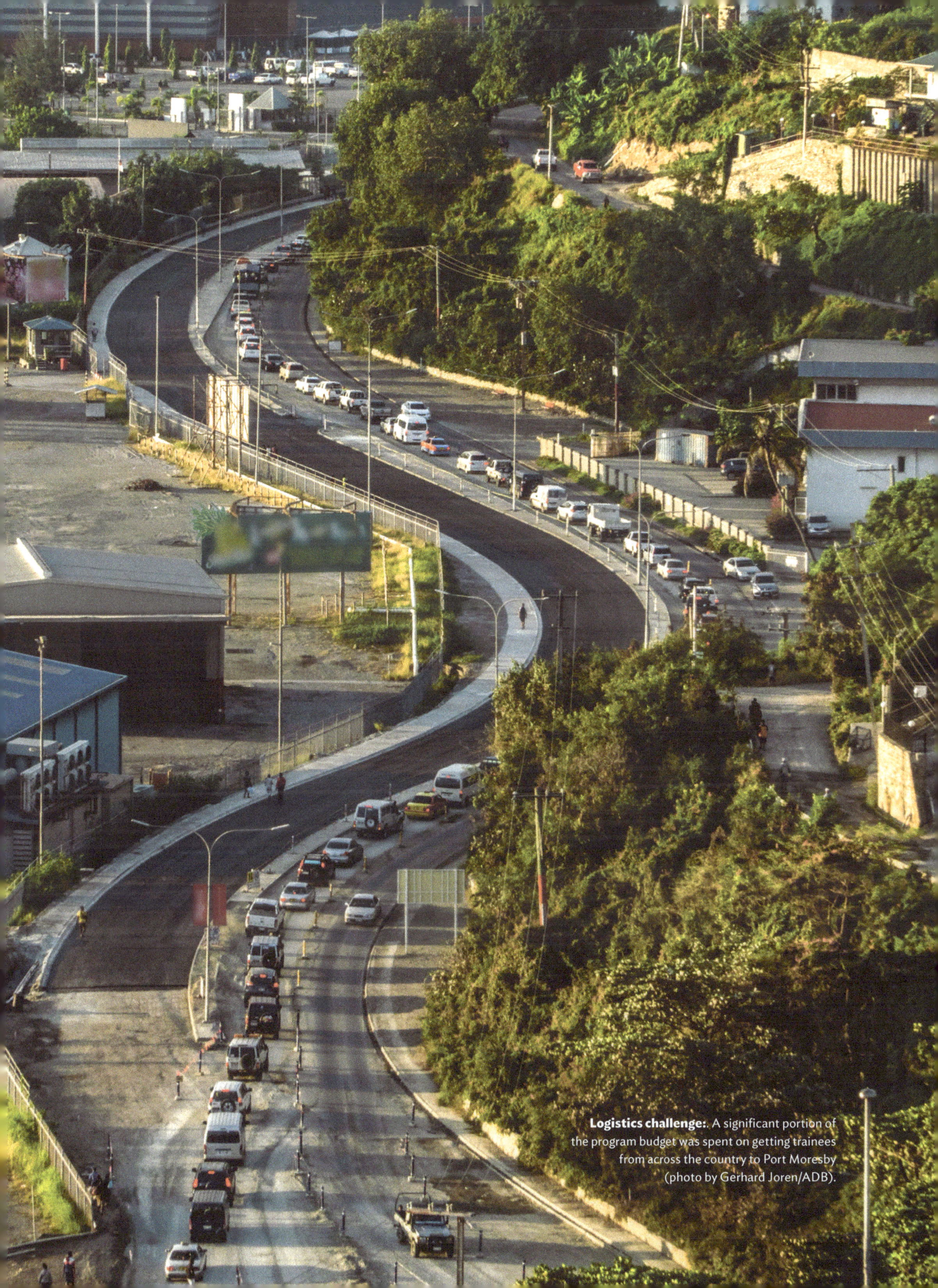

Logistics challenge:. A significant portion of the program budget was spent on getting trainees from across the country to Port Moresby (photo by Gerhard Joren/ADB).

www.ingramcontent.com/pod-product-compliance
Lightning Source LLC
Chambersburg PA
CBHW041800220926
51847CB00014B/267
9789292776626